CLINICAL PSYCHIATRY IN PRIMARY CARE

SECOND EDITION

Reviewers' Comments on First Edition

"For twenty years, I have been teaching psychiatry to nonpsychiatrist physicians and medical students. I have used a variety of texts, none of which have been very helpful for either theoretical understanding or practical interventions. This book, with its unique format and very practical content, is the finest book that I have had the opportunity to read. Those of us on the interface between psychiatry and medicine are indebted to the authors for this fine effort."

John L. Lightburn, M.D.
Associate Clinical Professor
of Family Practice & Psychiatry
University of Colorado Medical Center,
Denver, Colorado

"This book presents a highly useful approach to the evaluation and management of the common emotional and psychiatric problems seen by the generalist physician. I strongly recommend it to students, housestaff, and practicing physicians."

Paul Beck, M.D.
Associate Dean for Student Affairs
Associate Professor of Medicine
University of Colorado Medical Center,
Denver, Colorado

"A goldmine of useful advice and information."

The Lancet

"A probing, consciousness-raising manual which combines a unique format and relevant theoretical data."
Behavioral Medicine

CLINICAL PSYCHIATRY IN PRIMARY CARE

Second Edition

Steven L. Dubovsky, M.D.,

Associate Professor of Psychiatry
Associate Dean for Student Affairs

Michael P. Weissberg, M.D.

Associate Professor of Psychiatry
Director of Clinical Affairs

University of Colorado School of Medicine

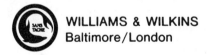

WILLIAMS & WILKINS
Baltimore/London

Copyright©, 1982
Williams & Wilkins
428 E. Preston Street
Baltimore, Md. 21202, U.S.A.

Made in the United States of America

Reprinted 1983, 1984

Library of Congress Cataloging in Publication Data

Dubovsky, Steven L.
  Clinical psychiatry in primary care.

  Includes bibliographies and index.
  1. Psychiatry. 2. Family medicine. I. Weissberg, Michael P. II. Title.
[DNLM: 1. Family practice. 2. Mental disorders. 3. Physician — Patient relations. 3. Psychopharmacology. WM 100 D818c]
RC454.D8 1982   616.89   82-1927
ISBN 0-683-02672-0   AACR2

Composed and printed at the
Waverly Press, Inc.
Mt. Royal and Guilford Aves.
Baltimore, Md. 21202, U.S.A.

To Mortimer H. Dubovsky, M.D.
and in memory of Gustav Weissberg, M.D.

PREFACE

We wrote the first edition of this book in the hope that it would provide a readable and practical guide to the management of psychiatric problems that are commonly encountered in medical practice. We have been gratified to learn that physicians in a wide spectrum of practices-- rural and urban, specialized and family practice--have found it useful. In this edition, we hope to provide an even more complete handbook for the clinician who must treat his patients' psychological and emotional, as well as their physical, problems. To accomplish this goal, we have rewritten the entire book and added a chapter on anxiety. All information on medications has been updated, and the reader will find new sections in each chapter, including sections on the identifi- cation of a functional somatic complaint, psychiatric effects of drugs used in medical practice, noncompliance and newer drugs used to treat depression.

Recently, a new diagnostic nomenclature has been introduced into psychiatric practice. This system, described in the 3rd edition of the <u>Diagnostic and Statistical Manual of Mental Disorders</u> (DSM-3), focuses on signs and symptoms of psychiatric disorders rather than presumed etiologies. DSM-3 diagnostic criteria are included throughout this volume.

A word about the print used in this book: As in the previous edition, we have attempted to avoid the expense of editing and type- setting by reviewing the manuscript ourselves and utilizing photo- offset rather than printing. We have attempted to choose the most appealing type and lettering, and hope that the reader will forgive the occasional typographical error that may have escaped our scrutiny.

Denver, Colorado
October, 1981

Steven L. Dubovsky, M.D.
Michael P. Weissberg, M.D.

ABOUT THE AUTHORS

Steven L. Dubovsky, M.D. is Associate Professor of Psychiatry and Associate Dean for Student Affairs at the University of Colorado School of Medicine. Dr. Dubovsky consults extensively to physicians in all specialties and sees patients with medical and psychiatric problems in his own practice. He has published original research in psychosomatic medicine as well as numerous articles and book chapters on the psychiatric aspects of medical practice. His most recent contribution is Psychotherapeutics in Primary Care.

Michael P. Weissberg, M.D. is Associate Professor of Psychiatry and Director of Clinical Affairs for the Department of Psychiatry of the University of Colorado School of Medicine. He is involved in the undergraduate, postgraduate and continuing education of physicians in many specialties and health professionals in many disciplines both within Colorado and throughout the United States. He has written numerous articles and book chapters on emergency psychiatry and the psychiatric aspects of medical practice.

ADDITIONAL CONTRIBUTIONS BY

Stephen L. Dilts, Ph.D., M.D. is Associate Professor of Psychiatry and Associate Director of Psychiatric Services at Denver General Hospital, where he supervises the treatment of large numbers of alcoholic and drug abusing patients.

Daniel A. Hoffman, M.D. teaches in the Sexual Dysfunction Clinic of the Department of Psychiatry of the University of Colorado School of Medicine, where he is a Clinical Instructor.

Ruth Fuller, M.D. is Assistant Professor of Psychiatry and Director of the Day Treatment Unit of the Department of Psychiatry of the University of Colorado School of Medicine. She is a practicing psychoanalyst with extensive experience treating families and couples in the public as well as the private sector.

ACKNOWLEDGMENTS

We will always be indebted to Peg Robbins for her support and dedication in producing a high quality book. We are also grateful to Maxine Peterson for her ongoing assistance and to Elaine Steffen for the long hours she worked to help us to meet our deadline.

Carol T. Stewart, M.D. was crucial to the development of the first edition of this book, and Dr. Michael Solomon contributed to the chapter on family problems. Richard Evans helped us to choose a presentable typeface and printed the chapter headings and sections of the chapter on reactions to illness and emergencies.

Tom Manoff, of the Manvo Institute, has continued to be a vital guiding force in conceptualizing our thoughts and developing the format for this book.

CONTENTS

1 HYPOCHONDRIASIS 1

The diagnosis and management of hypochondriacal
inpatients and outpatients is discussed, with
guidelines for starting medications or continuing
medications the patient is already taking.
Strategies for long-term treatment are developed.
Differentiation from other conditions which may
present with somatic complaints, especially
depression, is outlined. The identification of
the patient with a functional somatic complaint
is described.

2 DEPRESSION 24

New diagnostic schemes for depression are described,
and the diagnosis and treatment of depressed outpatients is outlined. The uses of psychotherapy
and antidepressant medication are described in
detail. Guidelines for the use of lithium are
provided, and other somatic treatments of affect
disorders are outlined in tabular form. The
evaluation of suicide potential and the management
of patients who have suicidal thoughts are
described in detail.

3 ANXIETY 57

The ways in which this ubiquitous problem may
present to the primary physician are described,
as is the psychological and pharmacologic approach
to types of anxiety that may interfere with a
patient's adaptation to a medical illness.
Diseases that present with anxiety are discussed.

who have made a suicide attempt, abusive
parents and spouses, and incest and rape
victims. The emergency management of these
conditions is described. Techniques for
restraining agitated patients and for keeping
patients in the hospital against their will
are outlined, as is emergency tranquilization.

INTRODUCTION

Most physicians encounter patients in their practices who have psychiatric problems that complicate or overshadow their medical or surgical illnesses. This book is a practical guide to the management of these patients.

The decision to cover the topics presented here was made after a literature search and a survey of practicing physicians throughout the United States made it evident that a relatively small number of psychiatric problems often is encountered by physicians who do not always feel equipped to deal with them. These problems include hypochondriasis and multiple somatic complaints, depression, anxiety, organic brain syndromes, alcohol and drug abuse, sexual problems, family problems, and complications of reactions to medical and surgical illnesses. While schizophrenic patients are not seen routinely by most physicians who do not practice psychiatry, their management often requires disproportionately great amounts of time. Since psychiatric emergencies are frequently encountered by house officers and by physicians who do not have readily available psychiatric backup, their management also was included.

The format of this manual reflects the doctor-patient interaction: Before devising an effective treatment plan, the physician must contend with his reaction to his patient. The doctor's reaction and its management therefore is the first topic in each chapter. Most clinicians try out approaches which seem to make sense before they finally develop a successful course of action, and learn about working with people through this trial and error method. The sections on unsuccessful and successful approaches provide this learning experience. If the reader understands the reasons why one approach does not work while another is successful, he will have mastered the psychodynamics of the problem under discussion. Because theoretical material is discussed in a clinical context, its usefulness will immediately be appreciated. Practical guidelines to the use of medications and psychotherapy, and of special problems appropriate to the problem being considered are discussed after general principles of treatment have been established. The differential diagnosis of each problem is considered when the reader thoroughly understands the condition. A consideration of the ways in which the psychiatrist may be helpful to the physician is provided at the end of each chapter. Only well-written review articles are included in the references.

Where appropriate, each chapter contains a section on practical psychopharmacology that provides guidelines for the prescription of psychotropic drugs. While doses and routes of administration are derived from our own experience and that of our colleagues, and from a review of the pertinent literature, the reader should thoroughly familiarize himself with the medications described before prescribing them.

This book may be read in its entirety, or the reader may wish to refer to sections of individual chapters. Each section is self-contained to permit easy references when the physician encounters the problems described in them. We are confident that our book will be clinically relevant, no matter how the reader wishes to use it.

Steven L. Dubovsky, M.D.
Michael P. Weissberg, M.D.

Chapter One

HYPOCHONDRIASIS

Hypochondriasis refers to a preoccupation with a real or imagined physical disorder that is greatly in excess of the disability that might be expected from the actual degree of physiologic disturbance. The patient focuses mainly on his symptoms and is impervious to the most convincing demonstrations that he has little or nothing to worry about. In fact, he exhibits remarkable "illness-claiming behavior": in the absence of objective pathology, the patient insists on being thought of as sick, and much of his behavior is directed toward proving this notion. Complaining about his illness occupies much of the patient's time and energy, and he seems determined to demonstrate his suffering to others. "Doctor shopping", on the surface, appears to represent an attempt to find a physician who can cure him. However, when one of his physicians attempts to make him feel better, the patient either gets worse or changes doctors again. He has a tremendous affinity for medications which, while ineffective in ameliorating symptoms, are extremely difficult to reduce or discontinue.

The hypochondriacal patient often appears in the hospital after a period of improvement or after his doctor has attempted to change his treatment regimen. He is accompanied by a thick chart and a litany of complaints, as if he feels the need to prove to his ward doctors how really sick he is. Although the patient may be under obvious psycho-social stress, he vigorously denies being concerned about anything except his illness and is angered when psychiatric consultation is called.

Not everyone with excessive physical complaints is a hypochondriac. Many individuals demonstrate increased somatic concerns in reaction to stressful situations. An obvious example is the previously healthy middle-aged man who has a myocardial infarction and temporarily becomes worried about a variety of symptoms that he fears may signal impending decompensation. Another is the medical student who reads about an illness and becomes convinced that he has it. Such "reactive hypochondriasis" is acute, occurs in response to stress and is reversible, responding positively to reassurance. While true hypochondriasis often appears after a mild illness, it is chronic and pervasive, and is unresponsive to, or gets worse with, reassurance.

The syndrome of "true" or "essential" hypochondriasis also is to be distinguished from a number of other disorders that may present with multiple and chronic somatic complaints, such as depression, hysteria, some psychoses, and organic brain disease. Somatic complaints are secondary to a disturbance of thinking or feeling in these conditions, while in true hypochondriasis somatic complaints are long-standing and play a central role in organizing the patient's life. The patient's need to be considered sick, illness-claiming behavior, characteristic response to treatment, and lack of awareness of the significance of his behavior also distinguish hypochondriasis from other psychiatric conditions.

CLUES TO THE DIAGNOSIS OF HYPOCHONDRIASIS

The presence of some or all of the following raises the suspicion of hypochondriasis:

1. Chronic complaints in one or more organ system that are out of proportion to demonstrable organic disease

2. Illness-claiming behavior

3. History of doctor shopping

4. History of medications or procedures working for a while, with an eventual return of symptoms

5. Reluctance to relinquish medications even when they do not help

6. Feelings in the physician of frustration, helplessness, and anger with the patient, accompanied by a wish to get rid of him

7. Negative response to reassurance (complaints continue or increase)

8. Negative response to abrupt changes in the treatment regimen (e.g., discontinuing medications, seeing the patient less frequently)

9. Positive response to acknowledgement of the severity of the patient's illness (complaints decrease or at least stabilize)

10. Positive response when the physician arranges for ongoing regular followup

11. Forceful denial of possible contributions of emotional factors to physical symptoms

12. Absence of other psychiatric illness

ENCOUNTER WITH A TYPICAL PATIENT

Mr. H. is a 45-year-old man who has been admitted to the hospital for further workup of back pain. A transcutaneous nerve stimulator was applied several months ago, producing some relief. When it stopped working, the patient's neurosurgeon felt that he had nothing more to offer and referred him to his current physician. The patient's pain increased progressively, and he was hospitalized in an attempt to carry out further diagnostic studies and achieve better control of his discomfort.

Mr. H. says that he was in good health and working as a truck driver until six years ago, when he wrenched his back while moving a piano. Following his injury he was off the job for a few weeks, after which his doctors advised him to return to work. However, each time he tried to return to work his back pain became so severe that he had to stop. About four years ago, Mr. H. developed another pain which would "be all over my head" and "would sometimes shoot down my back", and which has worsened over the years. He also complains of bloating and pain in his stomach, which he says are due to a hiatal hernia. He has had many treatments for his pain, including a back brace, various exercises, and numerous medications. He now takes Darvocet N-100, Tylenol with Codeine, Valium, an ergot preparation, and Maalox. Each treatment has seemed to work for awhile, only to lose its effectiveness. Similarly, each of the patient's numerous hospitalizations initially resulted in improvement, but was followed by a recurrence of symptoms. He now spends a good deal of his time in bed or visiting his doctors, and although he does not look incapacitated, he says he has been suffering constantly.

Pertinent past history includes the fact that Mr. H. was the youngest of four children who were raised by his mother after the patient's father died when the patient was three. His mother had to work most of the time to support the children, despite severe chronic arthritis, and the patient helped to care for the other children from the time he was six years old.

A thorough workup indicates that there is no new organic disease that might explain Mr. H's symptoms. When the doctor approaches Mr. H. to tell him the good news, the following conversation occurs:

Dr: We've gone over your tests carefully, Mr. H., and I'm pleased to tell you that your myelogram was normal.

Pt: Are you sure? I'm in an awful lot of pain. A few years ago the doctors at the other hospital said that I have an abnormality of my spine.

Dr: You are referring to a normal variation.

Pt: Yes, but not many people have the kind of pain that I have. It's killing me. I have chest pain too, and it goes into my stomach. Was my EKG normal?

Dr: That was normal, too. You really have nothing to worry about, so why not relax?

Pt: It's hard to relax when your health is so bad. My other doctors told me that I have a serious problem in the spinal cord--don't you think that we should get a CAT scan?

Dr: A CAT scan really wouldn't tell us much.

Pt: Then what sort of test should we order?

Dr: I don't really think that any more tests are indicated right now.

Pt: But what about my pain?

Dr: Let's talk about it later, OK?

THE PHYSICIAN'S REACTION TO HIS PATIENT

Physicians' reactions to their patients can be useful tools in making diagnoses and planning treatment. The comments in the right-hand column elucidate the kinds of information that can be obtained from the doctor's examination of his own feelings.

Physician's Reaction	*Comment*
Lack of awareness of any reaction	It would be unusual not to have a reaction to a patient who questions the physician's competence and seems inclined to direct his treatment in such an inappropriate manner. The absence of a conscious reaction under these circumstances usually indicates that the doctor is ignoring another feeling, often anger or frustration
Conviction that the physician is the only doctor who can help the patient	A feeling that the physician can produce miraculous improvement may represent the physician's attempt to overcome a sense of helplessness and a response to that part of the patient that stimulates rescue fantasies. If it is combined with an attraction to or unusual interest in the patient, this kind of reaction may indicate that the patient reminds the doctor of someone he once knew and liked. In either case, the physician is likely to become disappointed and angry when the patient does not improve
Impatience and a conviction that if the patient needs anything, it is a psychiatrist who can deal with his psychogenic problems	It is true that Mr. H. has a "psychogenic" problem. However, because he believes that his problems are organic, he will refuse to cooperate with any treatment plan that begins by telling him that his problems are "all in his head" and may leave the hospital if the physician insists that he acknowledge psychological problems immediately. (While some house officers might be relieved if the patient did leave, he is almost certain to return with increased complaints)

Physician's Reaction	*Comment*
Suspicion that an organic illness has been missed and desire to proceed with further diagnostic tests	When they are uncertain how to proceed, most people do what they know best. The physician who feels nonplussed by the patient therefore may proceed as though the patient had a disease that he knows how to treat
Frustration and anger	Most physicians would be inclined to feel angry with a patient who seems so unappreciative of his efforts. The self-pitying, demanding, dependent, hostile nature of the patient's interaction with the physician adds to the clinician's frustration and anger. These emotions are notoriously difficult to control

Frustration with hypochondriacal patients commonly results in:

1. Refusing to be "manipulated" and underprescribing medications

2. Overcompensating by "giving in" to the patient and prescribing unnecessary medications

3. Excess "professionalism" and aloofness in the service of ignoring the patient

4. Performing numerous unnecessary laboratory tests to prove that the patient is not really sick

5. Referring the patient to another service or physician

If he neither ignores nor acts on them, awareness of the doctor's reactions to the patient is helpful in making a diagnosis. Feelings in the doctor of frustration, helplessness, anger and a wish to get rid of the patient, or to force him to improve, are suggestive of hypochondriasis in the patient.

COMMON UNSUCCESSFUL APPROACHES

Skill in treating hypochondriacal patients can be increased when the physician understands approaches that are likely to be unsuccessful. Following are some commonly utilized approaches, along with the responses they are likely to provoke. The far-right column explains the patient's behavior.

Physician's Approach	*Patient's Response*	*Explanation*
Attempt to convince the patient that there is nothing physically wrong, for example, by showing him his lab test results, x-rays, or cardiogram	The patient finds some fault with the results he is shown, demands additional tests, or acknowledges that the organ system tested is normal but develops new symptoms	Telling the hypochondriacal patient that he is not ill is not reassuring to him because one purpose served by his symptoms is to convince the world (and himself) that he really is sick. This enables him to justify his seeking care-taking relationships with physicians. The prospect of not being considered ill threatens him with the loss of that care
Talk with the patient about the "emotional component" of his illness, and suggest that he see a psychiatrist	Some patients agree to see a psychiatrist to please their own doctor. However, they may do so with the unconscious intention of proving that a psychiatrist cannot help them. Many truly hypochondriacal patients openly refuse to see a psychiatrist, and respond to the suggestion of referral with an	The hypochondriacal patient does not know how to express "feelings" as anything but physical sensations, as if he had a defect in the part of his mind that experiences and deals with emotions. Forcing him to confront his emotions may impose a task he cannot handle, provoking anxiety that, like other distress, is

Physician's Approach	_Patient's Response_	_Explanation_
	increase in complaints in an attempt to prove that their problem is physical and not mental	expressed in somatic terms. Also, even if the physician does not imply that the patient's complaints are not "real", the patient may feel that the doctor is trying to "dump" him on the psychiatrist (which may be an accurate perception)
Engage in a search for the patient's alleged illness by ordering further tests	The patient improves temporarily when he feels that he is being taken seriously but develops new symptoms when one result is borderline abnormal	When all of the patient's and the physician's efforts are directed toward an illness that does not exist, little opportunity is provided to examine real psychosocial forces that influence the patient, and the patient's preoccupation with bodily function is reinforced. In addition, since all tests have a chance of showing some slight variation from normal, new tests may provide a focus for new symptoms
Change to another drug, for example, a stronger analgesic, to control the patient's pain	The patient's symptoms improve temporarily. However, even though the medication eventually becomes less effective, the patient refuses to discontinue it	Most new medications result in a temporary positive placebo effect. However, discontinuing the drug threatens the patient with the loss of another "badge of illness"

Physician's Approach	*Patient's Response*	*Explanation*
		Medications, as tangible evidence of the doctor's caring for the patient, acquire such importance to the patient that it is difficult to stop them once they are begun
Have the patient seen by many consultants in an attempt to elucidate his problem more completely	The patient's complaints increase and become more complex	The patient feels that his claim to illness is being tested, and he attempts to demonstrate how sick he is to each consultant in turn. Then, as each consultant questions the patient and orders more tests, new symptoms are inadvertently suggested

A SUCCESSFUL APPROACH

Since the hypochondriacal patient feels worse when attempts are made to reassure him that he is not really sick and resists early attempts to convince him that he has a psychiatric problem, an approach in which his need to be considered ill is acknowledged must be applied:

Dr: Although your tests give us no cause for immediate concern, I realize that you are feeling very, very sick. You are suffering with a great deal of pain.

Pt: How can my tests be normal if I'm having so much pain?

Dr: Our tests cannot always measure a patient's true experience of pain.

Pt: You know, one of the other doctors told me that my pain is psychosomatic.

Dr: We doctors are interested in the total patient, and so eventually we'll have to think about the impact your life experiences have on your illness, just as

we would with any patient. But I know that when
you feel sick it's hard to think of anything but
the pain.

Hypochondriacal patients often feel out of control of their lives,
and to make themselves feel more powerful, may become experts at
defeating their doctors. When the doctor attempts to prove himself
right (e.g., about whether the patient is "really" ill) and the
patient wrong, he always loses the fight. This situation is avoided
when the physician allows the patient a graceful way out of the
argument over whether his symptoms are measurable.

Many physicians dislike the idea of agreeing with the patient's
claim that he really is sick, and some feel frustrated if nothing is
done to "cure" the patient. Early in treatment, however, it is
important to realize that the hypochondriac's disability is as real
as any chronically ill patients. Like the patient with a chronic
disease, his symptoms are controlled rather than cured. Hypochondriasis
represents an unconscious (outside of the patient's awareness)
solution to a number of problems. It cannot willfully be turned on
or off, any more than can hallucinations, delusions, or compulsions.
Unconsciously, the patient cannot allow himself to get better, for
fear of having no other solutions to life's difficulties and no means
of excusing his failure to realize his potential in life. Treatment
in which more is expected of the patient than he is capable of
achieving increases his sense of being a failure and with it, his
complaints.

APPROACH TO DISCHARGE

COMMON UNSUCCESSFUL APPROACHES

Discharging a hypochondriacal patient from the hospital can be
a difficult task. Following are some commonly utilized approaches,
along with the reactions they are likely to provoke in the patient.
The far-right column explains the patient's response.

Physician's Approach	*Patient's Response*	*Explanation*
Tell the patient that since he is not sick enough to require further hospitalization he will be discharged and should	The patient appears in the emergency room with excruciating pain, demanding narcotics	Abruptly cutting the patient's connection to doctor and hospital frightens him. His anxiety is expressed by his

Physician's Approach	*Patient's Response*	*Explanation*
return if he experiences any further problems		physical complaints, which also express his anger at being abandoned by his doctors as well as his now intensified wish to be cared for by the hospital, a wish that the physician has told him can only be gratified if he develops further problems
Tell the patient that his emotions are affecting his complaints and that this situation is best treated by the psychiatrist	The patient replies that the only thing that is upsetting him is how much worse his pain has become: He now feels too sick to see a psychiatrist	The patient defends himself against the threat of not being thought to have a "bona fide" illness by increased attempts to prove that his illness is physical, not mental, and resists the threat of being abandoned by the psychiatrist by asserting his increased need for the primary physician
Point out that the patient is feeling better and no longer needs such intensive care	The patient's condition suddenly begins to deteriorate	In addition to the implication that he is no longer sick enough to require care, the patient's claim that he is suffering is challenged. Since many hypochondriacal patients have a need to display their misery in order to expiate a chronic sense of guilt, their demonstrations of pain and suffering tend to increase if they are not sufficiently unhappy to punish themselves

Physician's Approach	*Patient's Response*	*Explanation*
Inform the patient that he will be followed somehow after discharge but will be readmitted if his symptoms become disabling	The patient suffers increasingly disabling symptoms, necessitating rehospitalization	The implication that outpatient followup will be less satisfactory causes anxiety that results in increased complaints. By telling the patient how to get rehospitalized, the doctor guarantees that the patient's symptoms will indeed become disabling

A SUCCESSFUL APPROACH

Because he is chronically afraid of being abandoned, and because care seems guaranteed in the hospital, unless the patient is guaranteed meaningful followup, he is likely to resist discharge and seek rehospitalization. If the ward physician is unable or unwilling to provide ongoing assurance that the patient's needs will be met in the form of regular continuing contact with the doctor, he should arrange adequate followup by another physician to whom the patient is introduced while he is in the hospital:

Dr: Your case is very complicated, Mr. H. I'll need to follow you closely for some time.

Pt: Does that mean I should stay in the hospital until I feel better?

Dr: I know you want to get better quickly. However, you will probably have your symptoms for a while. The important thing now is that you have a doctor who is familiar with your case whether you're an outpatient or an inpatient.

Pt: But what if I get sicker?

Dr: The hospital always is available if you need it. But your status has to be monitored over time, and this can only be done on an outpatient basis. We don't expect you to be symptom-free before discharge.

Pt: But what about my medications? Does this mean
     you'll discontinue them?

Dr: We would need to discuss this issue thoroughly
     before deciding on any changes. Until I get to
     know you better, let's keep things the way they are.

OUTPATIENT MANAGEMENT

The hypochondriacal patient was forced to assume an adult role at
an early age because he had to take care of a sick parent, because one
parent was out of the home or because financial or other hardships made
normal parental caretaking relatively unavailable. As a result, the
patient became hyperindependent at an early age, at the expense of an
awareness of normal dependency needs, which became abnormally powerful
because they were never gratified. In later life, these needs are met
by being cared for by a physician, for a "bona fide" (to the patient)
illness, in imitation of a relative who received caretaking by being
sick. Since the patient does not consciously believe that it is right
to be dependent and remains unaware that he is looking for the care he
never received as a child, his symptoms provide a means by which he
has to be cared for. In addition to saying, "if not for my illness
I'd be more independent," the patient's symptoms excuse his failure to
achieve more in life, express hostility at parental stand-ins
(physicians) for not meeting his needs, punish himself for his anger
and his dependency, and control people he would otherwise feel helpless
to influence.

Most true hypochondriacs are unable to forego the use of somatic
complaints to adapt to the requirements of their internal and external
worlds. Once the legitimacy of their claim to illness is recognized,
less effort is expended attempting to convince the physician that they
are sick and their demanding, complaining behavior gradually decreases.
The goal of long-term management is to maintain their level of disability
at the lowest level that will allow them to function as best they can.
The following guidelines are useful in achieving this goal:

1. Tell the patient that he will probably always be ill,
   even though he may feel somewhat better at times.

2. Set regular appointments with the patient which he is
   expected to keep regardless of his state of health.
   He then will not have to feel sick in order to see
   the doctor.

3. Adopt a tolerant attitude toward the patient's symptoms, acknowledging his discomfort and suffering without promising relief.

4. Listen attentively if the patient begins to talk about the relationship between events in his life and the status of his symptoms. However, do not become too enthusiastic about his psychological-mindedness and allow the patient to return to his physical complaints. Gradually, he may be able to spend more time discussing his emotional problems if this does not result in loss of the sick role and access to his physician.

5. Tell the patient that, while the physician will respond to his symptoms promptly, repeated emergency calls will preclude good long-term care.

6. Periodic rehospitalization may be necessary, especially at times of emotional stress, to provide support and reassure the patient that his symptoms are considered "real". These admissions usually are provoked by an increase in complaints or other signs of panic. On admission, set a discharge date that is not contingent on the patient being symptom-free to teach the patient that, while the doctor takes his symptoms seriously, he will not permit the patient's symptoms to keep him in the hospital indefinitely.

7. When the doctor-patient relationship is solidified, appointments gradually may be made less frequent. Hypochondriacal patients in long-term treatment can be seen just a few times a year for 15 minutes or so, as long as another appointment is scheduled at the time of each visit and ongoing access to the physician is assured.

8. Attempt to find something likeable about the patient, if only that he has struggled admirably against adversity. The more interesting the patient seems, the easier it will be to care for him.

9. Some patients eventually do well enough to be dis-charged from care. However, it is difficult to predict in advance which patients will be this fortunate. Therefore, if the physician is not prepared to offer long-term treatment, or if the

patient makes his life miserable, he should consider
transferring the patient to a physician who is
willing to work with him.

10. If the patient is receiving financial compensation
for his disability, it may be especially difficult
to effect improvement that would threaten the
patient's livelihood. The physician also may feel
very uncomfortable certifying for insurance or
other purposes that the patient "really" is ill.
Usually, however, the physician can honestly state
that the patient is truly incapacitated by his
illness even if the patient's "illness-claiming
behavior" is reinforced by financial gain. Psychiatric consultation can be very helpful in dis-
tinguishing the malingerer or patient with a
compensation neurosis from the hypochondriac whose
claims for disability payment are only one symptom
of his illness.

APPROACH TO MEDICATION

Few hypochondriacal patients appear in the physician's office or
hospital without a long list of drugs, many of which are taken in
idiosyncratic ways. Usually, several doctors over the years have
written a variety of prescriptions as a concession to constant demands or
in the hope that the patient will leave them alone. The patient, who
has difficulty giving up even one pill, adds these to his treatment
regimen without discontinuing medications he is already taking. The
physician who encounters such a patient for the first time often is
appalled by the drug combinations embraced by the patient, and his
first impulse is to discontinue them immediately. Before attempting
this, the doctor should realize that the hypochondriacal patient becomes
attached to his medications for several reasons:

1. The pill represents the doctor's concern for him
in a tangible form

2. Taking medicine is proof that the patient is really
sick. Who ever heard of a sick person who does not
take medicine?

3. The physical sensations produced by the pill (usually
side effects such as dry mouth, dizziness, etc.) may
be important to the patient as indications that something is happening to his body

4. The ritual of pill-taking organizes the patient's day and lends meaning to his life

5. By continuing to take medicine the patient is "forced" to continue his association with doctors in order to refill prescriptions and can avoid an awareness of <u>wanting</u> to see his physician

6. At the same time, medications can provide a means to defeat the doctor by proving that the doctor's tools (drugs) do not really work. By doing so, the patient attains a sense of importance and control

If the physician recognizes the importance of medications to the hypochondriac, he will realize that an attempt to discontinue them abruptly is likely to result in panic on the patient's part which, like all other forms of distress, is expressed as increased somatic complaints.

The following guidelines are helpful in managing the hypochondriacal patient's medications:

1. Do not "try out" a drug that could not be continued for a long period of time

2. When not clearly indicated for a medical condition (e.g., digitalis), new drugs should not be too potent. Some relatively safe drugs to prescribe when the patient demands a new medicine are antihistamines, water soluble vitamins, amino acids and mild laxatives. These should be prescribed in such a way as to make it clear to the patient that the physician takes them seriously

3. Avoid drugs that produce abstinence syndromes when withdrawn (e.g., barbiturates) and addiction (e.g., most narcotics). Minor tranquilizers such as diazepam and chlordiazepoxide are preferable to powerful antidepressants (e.g., imipramine), hypnotics (sleeping pills), and antipsychotic drugs

4. Change to another drug of similar potency when one drug stops working

5. When pain medications are indicated, offer them regularly to the patient, allowing him to refuse them if he is not in severe pain. Prescribing

analgesics "PRN for pain" encourages the patient to
express pain in order to get a pill and focuses his
attention on pain and its relief

6. Treat acute pain with adequate doses of strong anal-
    gesics (see pp 141). Warn the patient in advance
    about the dangers of addiction in anyone and switch
    to a milder drug as soon as the acute illness resolves

7. Do not discontinue immediately drugs to which the
    patient has a strong psychological attachment unless
    there is a strong indication to do so, e.g., the drug
    is potentially dangerous or will produce adverse inter-
    actions with other drugs. Withdrawal of unnecessary
    medications is more likely to be accomplished after
    the doctor-patient relationship has stabilized

8. To discontinue a medication, reassure the patient that
    other drugs will be substituted if necessary, and that
    he will still receive continued followup

9. If a particular drug is unacceptable for any reason,
    and this is not a disguised expression of dislike for
    the patient, tell him truthfully why it will not be
    prescribed. Then follow guideline No. 8 and be
    prepared for a period of increased symptoms

THE "FUNCTIONAL" SOMATIC COMPLAINT

The perception of even the most organically derived pain is colored
by the patient's emotional state: anxiety and depression generally
increase reports of pain, while a relative absence of emotional distress makes any pain more tolerable. Nevertheless, the question often
arises whether a complaint for which no organic etiology can be found
is a manifestation of emotional conflicts rather than an as yet
undiagnosed medical illness. The presence of the following suggests
either a psychogenic etiology of a somatic complaint or a good deal of
functional overlay superimposed on a physical malfunction:

1. Idiosyncratic, dramatic or bizarre descriptions of
    symptoms, e.g., "like being seared with hot coals"
    or "like my arm is being torn off"

2. Symptom onset in association with a significant
    event (e.g., symptom first appeared after a loss)

or emotion (e.g., symptoms are most prominent when the patient is angry)

3. Persistence of complaints despite adequate medical therapy.

4. Strong denial that the patient's mood affects his pain or that any problems of living exist

5. Resistance to attempts to explore emotional issues (since organically determined complaints do not arise to solve a psychic conflict, the physically ill patient can afford emotionally to acknowledge psychological problems)

6. New symptoms develop when the patient is otherwise improving

7. Eagerness on the patient's part to describe pain and suffering in great detail

8. Conviction that the physician will cure the patient through some miraculous treatment, especially surgery

9. Pain that is experienced with equal intensity in two bodily locations at the same time

10. Multiple complaints that have been present since adolescence

DIFFERENTIAL DIAGNOSIS

A common cause of unexplained somatic complaints is organic disease that has not yet been diagnosed. Unexplained physical symptoms also may accompany a number of psychiatric conditions. These disorders are considered below, opposite differentiating elements from the history or examination of the patient. If positive evidence for one of these does not exist, the possible existence of an undiscovered physical illness should be considered.

Psychiatric Diagnosis	*Salient Differentiating Features*
The patient with <u>organic brain disease</u> may distract himself from his cognitive deficits by focusing on minor abnormalities elsewhere in his body (see Chapter 4). Hypochondriacs may develop acute organic brain syndromes, often due to drug intoxications or adverse interactions	-Disorientation to time and place -Short-term memory deficit -Attention disturbance -Special tests reveal cognitive dysfunction

Following the death of a loved one, patients experiencing <u>grief</u> may develop two types of somatic complaints:
  -Vague aches and pains (often headaches, backaches, tachycardia, indigestion and fatigue)
  -A symptom just like that experienced by the person who died (identification symptom), e.g., abdominal pain in the wife of a man who died of cancer of the stomach
	-History of recent loss or anniversary of loss
	-Signs and symptoms of grief (sadness, crying, preoccupation with the lost person)

Somatic complaints occasionally are an early sign of an <u>incipient psychosis</u>, usually schizophrenia. A delusional idea about the cause of the patient's symptoms usually is uncovered when he is asked why he thinks he is sick	-Unusual or bizarre thoughts -Hallucinations and delusions -Social withdrawal -Schneider first-rank symptoms -Inappropriate or flat affect -Impairment in ability to function -Odd or bizarre experiences, e.g, telepathy or communication with the dead
<u>Conversion Hysteria</u> is a rare condition, usually encountered on neurological services, in which an acute emotional	-Symptoms with symbolic meaning -Recent stress -Identification with a sick family member or friend

Psychiatric Diagnosis	*Salient Differentiating Features*
conflict is "converted" into a sensory or motor bodily symptom. Many patients labelled "hysterics" later are found to have true organic disease	-Past history of response to stress with somatic complaints -Secondary gain -Involvement of somatic nerves (voluntary nervous system and special senses) -Signs and symptoms accompanied by seeming unconcern about their significance ("la belle indifference")
Malingering is the conscious simulation of disease for financial or legal gain or to obtain drugs. It is uncommon in the average general hospital population	-Obvious significant gain that usually becomes obvious when the question, "What will happen if we keep the patient in the hospital?" is considered (usually avoiding jail or obtaining drugs or a large amount of money) -History of antisocial behavior or drug addiction -Onset before age 15 of truancy, expulsion from school, delinquency, persistent lying, fighting, promiscuity and running away from home
Anxiety, when accompanied by physiologic arousal, commonly produces signs and symptoms caused by hyperventilation and increased sympathetic activity. The patient may not be aware that he is anxious	-Obvious anxiety -Hypervigilence -Irritability -Motor tension -Multiple signs of sympathetic overactivity
Munchausen's syndrome (factitious disorder) is a rare condition in which the patient consciously simulates organic disease for the sole purpose of becoming a patient. Munchausen's patients are thought to have an underlying psychosis with unknown characteristics	-Improbable medical history -Appearance in the middle of the night for treatment of a chronic problem -Unavailable medical records -Hospitalizations under different names -Discharge against medical advice when the patient's symptoms are confronted or a psychiatrist is called

HYPOCHONDRIASIS VS. DEPRESSION

Depression (see p. 50) can be particularly difficult to distinguish from hypochondriasis when the depressed patient withdraws interest from the outside world and focuses it on his own body. This increased attention to minor somatic dysfunction results in somatic complaints, which can be chronic in chronic depression. In "depressive equivalents," the patient has somatic complaints in the absence of an obviously depressed mood. Important features differentiating depression from hypochondriasis are:

Depression	*Hypochondriasis*
-Vegetative signs (e.g., sleep disturbance, appetite and weight change)	-No vegetative signs
-Diurnal variation of somatic symptoms (worse in the morning, better as the day goes on)*	-No diurnal variation of symptoms
-Sadness	-Worry and anxiety
-Recent loss (e.g., of health money, or person)	-Recent minor illness more likely than a loss
-Reluctance to pursue contacts with physicians	-"Doctor shopping"
-Self-criticism	-Criticism of physicians
-Reluctance to advertise complaints	-"Illness-claiming behavior" in which advertisement of complaints is prominent and the patient's
-Positive response to antidepressants	life revolves around his symptoms
	-Initial positive response to anti-depressants followed by return of symptoms

* Also may occur with some medical illnesses, e.g., cluster headaches

USE OF THE PSYCHIATRIST

The hypochondriacal patient is best managed by a primary physician who is a constant, reliable, supportive deliverer of care. However, the requirement that the physician be prepared to follow the patient indefinitely and support "sick" behavior, as well as the trying nature of the patient, make this a difficult task. The psychiatrist can help the primary physician in several ways:

The physician should <u>consult with a psychiatrist</u>:

1. To confirm the diagnosis

2. To discuss the treatment plan

3. If the treatment plan does not seem to be working

4. If the doctor's reaction to the patient is hindering effective management

5. If symptoms abruptly change

6. If symptoms become bizarre

7. If chronic depression may be present

The physician should <u>refer the patient to a psychiatrist</u> when:

1. An additional psychiatric disease (e.g., psychosis, severe depression) is present

2. The patient decides to give up hypochondriacal symptoms, begins to talk about emotional conflicts, and requests psychotherapy to solve long-term problems

3. The primary physician is unwilling to follow the patient himself

REFERENCES

Dewesbury AR: Hypochondriasis and disease-claiming behavior in
    general practice. J Royal Coll Gen Pract 1973;23:379

Dorfman W: Hypochondriasis revisited: A Dilemma and challenge to
    medicine and psychiatry. Psychosomatics 1975;16:14

Dubovsky SL: Psychotherapeutics in primary care. New York,
    Grune & Stratton, 1981. pp 152-182

Idzark S: A Functional classification of hypochondriasis with
    specific recommendations for treatment. South Med J 1975;68:1326

Kenyon FE: Hypochondriacal states. Brit J Psychiatry 1976;129:1

Lipsett DR: Psychodynamic considerations of hypochondriasis.
    Psychother Psychosom 1974;23:132

Pilowski I: A general classification of abnormal illness behavior
    Brit J Med Psychol 1978;41:131

Strain JJ, Grossman S (Eds): Psychological care of the medically ill.
New York, Appleton, 1976 pp 76-92; 93-107

Wooley SC, Blackwell B, Winget C: A learning theory model of illness
behavior. Psychosom Med 1978;40:379

Chapter Two

DEPRESSION

Depression is one of the most frequently encountered problems in family practice and the most common psychiatric problem. Up to 15-30% of the general population, 24% of hospitalized patients, and even more medial outpatients are depressed. Most of these patients visit the primary doctor rather than the psychiatrist, while only about 25% are treated by psychiatrists. About 70% of all prescriptions for anti-depressants are written by nonpsychiatric physicians.

Depression is different from the ordinary sadness experienced by most people at some point in their lives. For example, many younger physicians may remember experiencing feelings of sadness, loneliness, and worry when they first left home to go to college. Despite their discomfort, they continued to function, and their symptoms abated when the situation which caused them resolved (e.g., when the college student returns home for the summer). Although symptoms may return from time to time, they are generally short-lived and not too disabling, and human contact and reassurance make the patient feel better. Depression is distinguished from such normal "reactive sadness" by more severe, pervasive and disabling symptoms that continue after the stress that provoked them has abated. The patient may have reacted to similar stresses with depression in the past and may develop signs of biological dysfunction in addition to sadness.

Many patients complain of "feeling depressed", but not all are suffering from clinical depression. This diagnosis is associated with the presence of a cluster of signs and symptoms called the "depressive triad":

1. A pervasive disturbance of mood. The patient experiences sadness, crying, discouragement and irritability. Anxiety may accompany depressive feelings.

2. A disturbance in perception of the self, the environment, and the future. Negative expectations color the patient's perceptions of himself and his world. He may experience helplessness, hopelessness, a heightened sense of guilt, lowered self-esteem, loss of interest in usual activities (including sex) and feelings that life seems so miserable that death seems preferable and suicide a viable alternative.

3. Alterations in biological function (vegetative signs).
   A sleep disturbance, especially early morning awakening,
   may be present and this often is accompanied by a diurnal
   variation of symptoms (worse in the morning, better as the
   day goes on). Patients also may complain of an appetite
   disturbance and corresponding weight change (usually
   decreased), constipation, tachycardia, fatigue, agitation,
   difficulty concentrating, indecisiveness, multiple somatic
   complaints, and slowed thinking and behavior (psychomotor
   slowing).

Depression can be diagnosed when some of these symptoms have been
present for at least two weeks or when almost all, especially vegetative
changes, are obvious and severe.

Mania is the psychological and behavioral opposite of depression.
The patient is euphoric, expansive or irritable and exhibits increased
energy and activity, grandiosity, expansiveness, decreased need for
sleep, distractability, racing thoughts (flight of ideas) and pressure
to keep on talking (pressure of speech). He may spend money unwisely
and otherwise overestimate his capabilities and resources. Although
the patient may be humorous and cheerful, he responds to attempts to
calm him with anger and insults. If manic symptoms are not grossly
incapacitating, the patient is said to have hypomania.

Various classifications have been applied to depression. Commonly
used categories include:

1. Endogenous depression (melancholia). Symptoms do not appear
   in response to an obvious psychological precipitant or are
   greatly out of proportion to environmental events and last
   after external events have changed for the better. The
   patient does not respond positively to other people, and
   interpersonal therapies alone are not curative. Vegetative
   (biological) changes, are usually present, and the patient
   is likely to have a positive response to somatic treatments
   for depression (medications and electroshock therapy).
   Past history and family history often are positive for
   depression. A biological component is further suggested
   by the failure of 2/3 of patients with this diagnosis to
   supress serum cortisol production after being given
   dexamethasone (described further below).

2. Reactive depression. Symptoms appear in response to an
   obvious psychological precipitant. The patient is responsive
   to his environment, making psychological interventions more
   successful initially than in endogenous depression. Anxiety
   and agitation are more prominent than in endogenous
   depression, and response to somatic therapies is less
   predictable. Past history and family history often are
   negative for depression.

3. Neurotic depression. Symptoms interfere with some but not all areas of functioning and self-pity and irritability are prominent. Neurotic depression often is equated with reactive depression and with dysthymic disorder (see below).

4. Psychotic depression. Symptoms are extremely severe, with hallucinations, delusions, or gross incapacitation in most areas of function. Perhaps due to an increasing tendency to treat depression early, only about 10% of depressed patients are psychotic.

5. Involutional melancholia. Symptoms consist mostly of anxiety and somatic complaints, with an underlying severe depression. The course is prolonged and prognosis is poor. Involutional depression used to be a frequently made diagnosis in older patients (age 45-60); however, this diagnosis rarely is made today.

6. Chronic depression (dysthymic disorder). Although the majority of depressive episodes remit within 9 months to a year, 10-20% of acutely depressed patients do not recover completely. These patients' symptoms (primarily depressed mood, inability to enjoy life, loss of energy, decreased productivity, irritability, pessimism and self-pity) may lift for a few days to a month or two, but depressed feelings then return. The term "neurotic depression" has been replaced by "dysthymic disorder" in the current psychiatric nomenclature, although symptoms must be present for at least 2 years before this diagnosis can be made. Chronically depressed patients are at increased risk of developing physical illnesses, perhaps because they do not take care of themselves.

7. Masked depression. A depressed mood, of which the patient is unaware, is hidden by chronic somatic complaints such as back pain, headache, facial pain, arthralgias, and gastrointestinal complaints or by alcoholism and drug abuse.

8. Mixed anxiety and depression. Complaints of anxiety are prominent, and it may be difficult to determine whether the patient is anxious about being depressed or depressed because he is anxious.

A simpler means of classifying depression considers only whether depression is the only disturbance. According to this scheme, all depressions (diagnosed by the presence of the "depressive triad") are classified as:

1. Primary depression (primary affect disorder). Depressive
    symptoms occur in the absence of any other psychiatric,
    medical or surgical disorder. Primary depression is
    further subdivided into:

    -Unipolar depression (major depression). The patient
    experiences single or recurrent episodes of depression
    only. Patients often have a positive family history
    of depression and suicide, and sometimes of alcoholism
    and antisocial behavior, but a negative family history
    of mania.

    -Bipolar depression (bipolar illness or manic depressive
    disease). The patient has experienced at least one
    episode of mania or hypomania, with or without
    depression.

2. Secondary depression. Depressive symptoms occur in the
    context of a serious medical, surgical, or other
    psychiatric illness, even though they may be indistin-
    guishable from those of unipolar depression. Past and
    family history usually are negative for depression.

Theories of the etiology of depression have taken genetic, developmental,
biological, and psychological factors into account. For example, some
people seem to be genetically at risk of developing depression. These
patients have family histories of affect disorders (depression or mania),
and they may become depressed in the absence of an obvious psychological
precipitant. Indications of biological dysfunction (vegetative signs)
appear when they become depressed, and psychological interventions alone
seldom produce improvement. Disturbances in brain function have been
implicated in some of these depressions. Recent research has focused
on alterations in neurotransmitter metabolism in areas of the brain
thought to mediate reward and punishment: drugs that lower brain
concentrations of norepinephrine and serotonin, for example, reserpine,
can produce depression, while drugs that increase the concentrations
of these substances ameliorate depression. Also, concentrations of
metabolites of norepinephrine and serotonin in CSF and urine have been
found to be low in some patients suffering from depression and high in
those experiencing mania. Reversible changes in brain biogenic amine
homeostasis that are triggered by some drugs and illnesses, or that
occur spontaneously for unknown reasons, therefore, are thought to
produce one type of depressive state.

That some depressions are at least associated with, if not caused
by, a profound shift in neuroendocrine homeostasis is illustrated by
the recent finding that some depressed patients fail to suppress
cortisol production when challenged with an exogenous adrenal steroid.
While most normal individuals demonstrate lowering of serum cortisol on
the day after being given 1 mg of dexamethasone at 11 P.M., many

endogenously depressed patients maintain serum cortisol levels above 5 μg/dl, indicating hyperactivity of the pituitary-adrenal-cortical axis. In the absence of a medical illness that might affect this test, one can say with 92% confidence that a patient with an abnormal dexamethasone suppression test (DST) is endogenously depressed, even if the diagnosis is not clinically apparent. While there are few false positive results, more false negatives may occur.

Patients who are not genetically predisposed to depression may be sensitized to loss later in life if they have suffered the loss of a parent or other significant family member in childhood. These individuals, and people who have suffered other deprivations as children, may suffer a resurgence of earlier unresolved feelings of sadness, hopelessness and helplessness when they are confronted by setbacks later in life. While all people who experience childhood bereavement do not become depressed later on, the early loss of a parent or other childhood hardship is found frequently in depressed patients.

Many depressions appear in response to a loss. The kinds of losses, both symbolic and actual, that can precipitate depression include loss of an important relationship, health, body parts, status, self-esteem, attractiveness, attention from others, or financial security. A person may be psychologically sensitized to loss in a variety of ways:

1. He may have had an earlier important loss, e.g., death of a parent in childhood. A loss in the present reminds him of the past loss, and feelings surface that were buried but unresolved.

2. He may have had mixed feelings (ambivalence) about the lost person. If he learned as a child that expressing anger is wrong or bad, he may not permit himself to express or even to experience any anger he may have felt with the lost person (if only for leaving him). The patient then turns the anger against himself as a safer and more convenient target in the form of depression, at the same time punishing himself for having "bad" feelings.

3. He may depend excessively on people, strength, a job, attractiveness, etc. for self-esteem. Loss of the external source of self-esteem causes a loss of self-esteem in the patient as well, resulting in depression.

4. He may depend excessively on others for nurturing and caring, and feel that he cannot accomplish important goals without their support. When he loses a supportive relationship he feels incapable of accomplishing these goals and the resulting sense of helplessness produces depression.

Depression also may be learned. For example, repeated negative experiences from which the patient cannot escape may make him feel helpless to overcome adversity. Negative expectations that are learned in other situations may result in a self-fulfilling prophecy in which the patient becomes convinced that he cannot help himself, does not exert enough effort on his own behalf, fails, and becomes even more discouraged and depressed.

Understanding depression requires an awareness of the possible influences of psychological, behavioral, cognitive and biological variables. Interventions directed against disturbances in all areas then can be devised.

CLUES TO THE DIAGNOSIS OF DEPRESSION

1. Symptom duration of at least two weeks or very severe symptoms

2. Some or all of the symptoms of the "depressive triad":

    -Pervasive disturbance of mood; sadness, discouragement, crying, irritability, anxiety

    -Disturbance in perception of the self, the environment and the future: loss of interest in usual activities, helplessness, hopelessness, guilt, lowered self-esteem, decreased interest in sex, suicidal thoughts

    -Vegetative signs: behavioral slowing or agitation, sleep disturbance, diurnal variation, appetite and weight change, constipation, tachycardia, fatigue, somatic complaints, slowed thinking, difficulty concentrating, indecisiveness

3. History of a recent loss (of person, health, income, etc.)

4. Past history of depression and/or mania

5. Past history of response to antidepressant medications or ECT

6. Family history of depression, suicide, alcoholism, mania or antisocial behavior

7. Suicidal thoughts

8. Abnormal dexamethasone suppression test

ENCOUNTER WITH A TYPICAL PATIENT

Mrs. D is a 35-year-old married woman who was admitted to the hospital for a hysterectomy because of endometriosis. Surgery was uneventful, although post-operatively the patient seemed slow to ambulate. During her first follow-up visit, the patient complains of continued pain in the incision and trouble sleeping. The doctor reassures her that she is healing normally and continues the sleeping pill. Two months later, Mrs. D seems worried and has a downcast expression on her face. The following conversation occurs:

Dr: How have you been doing, Mrs. D?

Pt: Just fine...but I'm still having some pain. Could something have gone wrong with my surgery?

Dr: The pain should be much less by now.

Pt: Maybe it is a little. But it still seems to hurt. And I'm so tired all the time.

Dr: Have you been able to get back to work yet?

Pt: No...I don't have enough energy...I don't want to be any trouble, but I just don't feel right inside (starts to cry, then stops herself)... I'm sorry, I don't know what got into me.

Dr. That's OK. But you really don't have to worry. Your wound is healing well and you should be feeling better.

Pt: I suppose so...I don't know what's wrong with me (looks worried)

THE PHYSICIAN'S REACTION TO HIS PATIENT

Depressed patients often present with a mixture of irritability and sadness that may evoke strong feelings in the physician even before the patient's emotions become apparent. Common reactions are listed in the left-hand column below. The comments in the right-hand column further elucidate the physician's reaction.

Physician's Reaction	*Comment*
Inability to understand why the patient is so upset after a simple operation	Failure to understand the patient may indicate that the doctor is distracted by a strong feeling of his own. Physicians who have experienced depression themselves may find it particularly difficult to perceive depression in their patients. Uncertainty about how to help the patient also may lead the physician to fail to identify depression
Anger with the patient	The patient's failure to improve, questioning the doctor's competence, and failure to respond to reassurance are irritating. Irritation also may serve to turn the physician's attention away from the patient's sadness
Impatience for the interview to end	Discomfort arising from not knowing how to help the patient or difficulty tolerating depressive feelings may make the physician anxious to get her out of his office and may result in a failure to obtain sufficient information to make a diagnosis
Sadness	When the doctor does not avoid it by feeling puzzled or irritated, sadness is a common empathic response to the depressed patient. It may be accompanied by hopelessness about the patient's chances of recovery and worry that unless a specific medication is prescribed immediately, the patient cannot be helped

COMMON UNSUCCESSFUL APPROACHES

Because the depressed patient is sensitive to nuances in interpersonal relationships, the doctor's approach is crucial. Following
are some unsuccessful approaches physicians may use when working with
depressed patients, along with the patient's response and an explanation of the patient's behavior.

Physician's Approach	*Patient's Response*	*Explanation*
Attempt to cheer up or reassure the patient by telling her not to worry or to stop feeling sorry for herself	The patient's depression increases	Many depressed patients have a strong sense of guilt, and see the doctor's attempts to reason with them or force them to feel better as a criticism. If the patient could will herself to improve she would not be depressed; when she cannot, her feelings of failure and guilt increase, exacerbating her depression
Agree with the patient that her situation is hopeless	The patient becomes more depressed and develops suicidal thoughts	Even though she may express hopelessness, the depressed patient would not consult the physician if she did not also maintain some hope that someone may be able to help her. If this last remaining hope is undermined, the patient may feel she has nothing to live for

Physician's Approach	*Patient's Response*	*Explanation*
Attempt to take the patient's mind off her problems by changing the topic when she describes her sadness in detail	Although the patient stops talking about how depressed she feels, her complaints persist or increase	Although the patient attempts to cover up feelings that the physician does not seem to wish to discuss, she feels rejected and angry at not being understood, and expresses her disappointment as depression and failure to improve
Prescribe a month's supply of an anti-depressant and a sleeping pill, and offer to see the patient in a month	The patient overdoses on the medication the doctor prescribes	Many depressed patients feel worthless and uninteresting. Not arranging for close follow-up intensifies the patient's feeling that she is not worth the physician's interest, prevents her from meeting her need to depend on the physician (an important need which many depressed patients find it difficult to ask for openly), and makes it difficult for the physician to follow the patient closely enough to monitor suicide potential

A SUCCESSFUL APPROACH

When the patient expresses sadness and irritability, and the doctor finds himself feeling annoyed, put off, or overly pessimistic, it is possible that the patient is depressed. The next step is to help the patient to express underlying emotions so that the nature of the depression may be defined:

Dr: You seem very worried and sad.

Pt: I have been feeling a little sad...my husband says that I have been crying at night.

Dr: What goes through your mind when you cry?

Pt: Sometimes I wonder if there's something still wrong inside of me...whether I'm less of a woman since the operation...I wonder if my husband still loves me.

Dr: Why do you wonder that?

Pt: Because it seems that I must have done something wrong...I feel like I've been a bad wife and mother...

Dr: Do you have any hope that things will get better?

Pt: If you say so...

Dr: You don't seem so sure.

Pt: Well, I'm not sure anything will help...sometimes I don't think I'll ever get better.

The patient has described sadness, crying spells, lowered self-esteem, a heightened sense of guilt and hopelessness. To obtain a clearer picture of the patient's depression, the physician also should inquire about:

1. Other signs and symptoms of the depressive triad

2. Past history of depression

3. History of response to treatment for depression

4. Past history of mania or hypomania. The physician may ask, "Have you ever felt the opposite of the way you feel now; full of energy and very happy. Has there ever been a time when you needed little sleep, were more active than usual, and spent a lot of money?"

5. <u>Family history of depression, suicide, mania, alcoholism</u>
   <u>and antisocial behavior</u>

6. <u>Family history of successful treatment with anti-</u>
   <u>depressants or electroshock</u>

Once the diagnosis of depression is confirmed, the physician must evaluate <u>suicide potential</u>. This is a crucial element in the <u>routine</u> evaluation of <u>any</u> depressed patient. It is often mistakenly left out of a physician's initial workup for several reasons:

1. The physician may be afraid of putting the thought of suicide into the patient's head. However, the patient is unlikely to volunteer suicidal thoughts without being asked. If the patient has not thought of suicide he will say so unequivocally and will be relieved that the doctor cared enough to ask. It is impossible to make a patient feel suicidal by asking about the thought.

2. The doctor may feel that he would not know what to do if he found that the patient were suicidal. However, suicide is preventable, and much can be done to help the suicidal patient. In fact, the clinician's asking about suicide decreases the patient's sense of desperation and isolation, and is therapeutic in and of itself.

3. The physician may wish to deny the seriousness of the patient's depression by ignoring the possibility of suicide.

4. The clinician may be unaware of how common suicidal thoughts are in depressed patients. If the patient does not seem profoundly depressed, the physician may feel that the patient "is not depressed enough" to feel suicidal. However, suicide risk is not correlated with severity of depression.

5. The doctor may not know the correct questions to ask in order to elucidate the risk of suicide.

EVALUATION OF SUICIDAL POTENTIAL

Between 5 and 15% of depressed patients kill themselves! It is therefore imperative that the physician ask all depressed patients about suicide. Most patients who suicide are in contact with their primary physician shortly before their suicide, although they may not volunteer that they intend to kill themselves. If the physician asks a few pointed questions the plan can be uncovered, and steps to prevent death can be taken. If he does not, the patient is very likely to make a suicide attempt (in one study 55% of patients who died by overdose killed themselves with medication obtained in one prescription at their last visit to their doctors).

While many patients think about suicide for some time before killing themselves, the actual event often is impulsively carried out. If suicide is prevented, the patient almost invariably changes his mind about killing himself when his depression improves. It is the doctor's job to identify the patient at risk and to take steps to prevent suicide while depression is being treated.

The following guidelines will help the physician to identify the suicidal patient:

1. If the patient does not volunteer thoughts about suicide, ask: "Have you been feeling that life is not worth living?"

2. If the patient says yes, ask specifically: "Have you had thoughts of killing yourself?"

3. If the patient again says yes, ask: "What are your thoughts?"

4. If the patient does not volunteer a suicide plan, ask: "Do you have a plan to kill yourself?" If the answer is yes, determine whether the plan carries a high risk of lethality and whether it can be carried out. A patient who plans to shoot himself but has no gun is not in as immediate danger as the patient who is thinking of over-dosing and has medication as home that he plans to take when he leaves the doctor's office.

5. Inquire about rehearsal of the plan. The patient who has put a loaded gun to his head or stared longly at a bottle of pills in the medicine cabinet is likely to be preparing himself to die.

6. Ask: "What do you expect to happen if you kill youself?" The patient who says that he really does not expect to die is at less risk than the patient who has clear ideas about who will attend his funeral, how people will feel about him when he is gone, etc. The patient who makes a suicide attempt without planning to die can of course miscalculate and end up just as dead as the patient who fully intended to die all along.

7. If the physician is still unsure about the risk of
    suicide, evaluate factors that are associated with
    high suicide risk:

    -Past history of a suicide attempt, especially
     if it was serious, violent, carefully planned,
     or if two or more attempts were made

    -Presence of hopelessness

    -Family history of suicide

    -Social isolation and loneliness

    -Recent separation from a loved one, especially
     if no other emotional supports are available

    -Psychosis, especially with hallucinated voices
     telling the patient to kill himself ("command"
     hallucinations)

    -History of impulsive behavior

    -Chronic or terminal illness

    -Organic brain syndrome

    -Alcoholism or drug abuse

    -Withdrawal of family members from the patient

    -Covert or overt wish by a family member that
     the patient die

    -Older, single, male

    -Severe insomnia

8. Now the doctor must evaluate his own reaction to the patient.
    Does he _feel_ that the patient may be suicidal, regardless
    of the information already gathered? If so, that feeling
    should be taken seriously.

9. If suicide is a possibility, obtain immediate psychiatric
    consultation.

10. Since suicidal and homicidal thoughts frequently accompany
    each other, evaluate the suicidal patient's dangerousness
    to others (see p. 262).

SUBTLE CLUES TO SUICIDE

Some patients hint indirectly that they are thinking of killing themselves, hoping consciously or unconsciously that their plan will be uncovered. Behaviors or statements by patients that should alert the physician to hidden suicidal thoughts include:

1. Forceful denial or indignation in response to being asked about suicide

2. Making a will, giving away personal property, or otherwise setting affairs in order

3. Talking about taking a long trip

4. Asking the doctor to look after the patient's family

5. Complaining that nothing seems to be getting better

6. Preoccupation with death, e.g., wondering aloud what it would be like to be dead or repetitive dreams of death or injury

7. Preoccupation with a dead relative or friend

8. Sudden resignation and calm in a patient who has been protesting about how badly he feels, when there is no obvious explanation for his improvement

9. Any feeling on the physician's part that the patient may be suicidal

HOW TO PROCEED AFTER EVALUATING SUICIDE POTENTIAL

1. If the patient is in imminent danger of killing himself, he should be hospitalized on a medical or psychiatric floor immediately, and psychiatric consultation should be obtained (see pp. 270-71). Although it usually is reassuring to the patient, hospitalization alone does not eliminate the danger, and round-the-clock observation should be provided.

2. If the patient refuses voluntary hospitalization, the procedure described on pages 267-268 should be followed and involuntary admission obtained. The danger of a successful lawsuit is very slight if the physician acts in accordance with this procedure.

On the other hand, up to 15% of patients who kill themselves do so after being allowed to refuse hospitalization.

3. If the patient has thoughts about suicide but is certain that he will not act on tnem, at least in the near future, consult with a psychiatrist for help in evaluating this promise. Some of these patients may be followed as outpatients if the physician is certain that they will call if they begin to feel more suicidal and if he can provide close follow-up.

4. If suicidal thoughts are fleeting or absent, begin outpatient treatment. Re-evaluate suicide potential if the patient gets worse, does not improve, or develops any of the subtle signs listed above.

5. Instruct the patient to call at any time if suicidal thoughts develop or if distress increases.

APPROACH TO PSYCHOTHERAPY

While medications are an important part of the therapeutic approach to the depressed patient, many depressions arise in the context of an important relationship, and an interpersonal approach can be very useful in correcting distorted feelings and attitudes. Contact with the physician replaces the relationship whose actual or threatened loss has precipitated or exacerbated depressive feelings. The doctor then is able to help the patient's feelings to seem more manageable and less frightening by putting them into words:

Dr: Your sadness, along with the other symptoms we discussed are symptoms of the kind of depression that is likely to respond to medications and to our talking about your emotions.

Pt: How can talking about my feelings possibly help?

Dr: I know that you feel pessimistic about the possibility of any treatment helping you. However, that feeling, too, is a symptom of your depression and we're lucky because your depression can be treated and you will feel better. We'll start by trying to figure out why you became so depressed. I want you to plan on meeting with me in two days, when we'll have enough time to start talking about this. Then I want to see you regularly, for about 20 minutes per visit.

If anything comes up before your next appointment, I want you to call me. Don't hesitate
to call any time, day or night.

Pt: Do you think it will help? What if I don't get better?

Dr: You are suffering from a condition with a very high
cure rate and you'll find that my treatment is
very likely to work.

The physician's interest in and acceptance of the patient helps
her to feel that, since an important person--her doctor--thinks she is
important enough to meet with regularly, she is not so worthless. By
making regular appointments he legitimizes her need to depend on him,
and supplies a shared future that contains the hope for improvement.

Some physicians have the impression that it requires great skill to
talk to depressed patients. However, in uncomplicated depressions that
represent a psychobiological reaction to a life stress, understanding
how the patient's emotions and thinking have caused the depression and
pointing out inappropriately negative expectations can be enormously
helpful. If the patient can be induced to verbalize these emotions and
thoughts, steady support and reassurance from the doctor may help the
patient to find a more adaptive solution to the problem that has caused
him to feel depressed. This can be successfully accomplished with a
psychological approach utilizing short (about 20 minute) interviews
once or twice a week. Psychotherapy facilitates, and is facilitated by,
the appropriate use of medications. This approach should be applied
to patients who:

1. Do not present a severe risk of suicide or homicide

2. Are not psychotic

3. Are responsive to the physician's comments

4. Have a depression that appeared in response to a
   psychological stress

5. Do not have a history of impulsive, violent or
   self-destructive behavior

6. Have at least one supportive relationship

7. Have a past history of a good response to
   psychotherapy

Treating depression with psychotherapy involves the application of the following techniques:

1. Establishing and maintaining a positive, supportive, relationship

2. Maintaining a hopeful attitude

3. Setting regular appointment times, informing the patient in advance how long each appointment will last

4. Remaining available to the patient at all times during the acute phase of the illness: If the patient feels confident that the doctor really is available he is unlikely to need to test the physician's availability with repeated calls or complaints

5. Encouraging the patient to express emotions and unburden himself of them

6. Defining the problem to make it more manageable and enable the patient to gain some intellectual control of his situation. A situation that is obvious to the physician (e.g., that the patient is responding to the loss of her uterus) may not be at all obvious to the patient

7. Clarifying feelings and thoughts, thereby making them easier to manage, e.g., "You mean that you feel less attractive without a uterus"

8. Confronting aspects of reality that the patient seems to ignore, e.g., "You seem more than a little depressed"

9. Interpreting meanings that are beyond the patient's immediate awareness, thereby helping her to make connections of which she was previously unaware, e.g., "Perhaps you feel your husband will leave you for a more attractive woman"

10. Setting realistic goals that the patient can accomplish without fear of failure

11. Maintaining a hopeful attitude that problems can be faced and dealt with more effectively

12. Remaining alert to the possibility of suicide

APPROACH TO MEDICATION

Many patients with depressive symptoms improve after a few visits or with a change in their external environment (e.g., a reconciliation with a spouse whose departure precipitated depression) and do not need an antidepressant. These patients can be seen a few times without prescribing a drug in order to determine whether psychotherapy alone will work. If insomnia is a problem during this exploratory phase a sleeping medication (e.g., flurazepam) may be used.

Severe depressions associated with biological dysfunction (as indicated, for example, by vegetative signs) are thought to be associated with alterations in brain neurotransmitters that may be improved by somatic therapies (medications and, in more severe cases, electroshock). Conditions under which somatic treatments should be considered include:

1. Vegetative signs (e.g., anorexia, significant weight loss, early morning awakening and diurnal mood swing) have been consistently present

2. There is a past history of response to a somatic treatment

3. Family history is positive for depression

4. There is a family history of good response to somatic treatment for depression

5. Symptoms are severe

6. Psychotic symptoms (e.g., hypochondriacal delusions such as "my body is riddled with cancer" or delusions of guilt or sin) are present

7. Symptoms did not appear in response to an obvious precipitant

8. The patient does not respond to psychotherapy

9. The patient has an abnormal dexamethasone suppression test (1 mg. of dexamethasone is given orally at 11 PM, and blood is drawn at 4 PM and 11 PM the next day. Serum cortisols greater than 5, and probably 4, μg/dl indicate failure of suppression of cortisol production)

Most somatic therapies for depression are thought to produce improvement by increasing available norepinephrine (and possibly serotinin) at synapses in "reward centers" in the brain. Tricyclic and tetracyclic antidepressants block reuptake of these "biogenic amines" into the presynaptic axon, and monoamine oxidase (MAO) inhibitors interfere with their degradation by the enzyme MAO. Electroshock therapy (EST or ECT) is thought to increase available central biogenic amines by an unknown mechanism. Phenothiazines (especially thioridazine) can produce improvement in depression associated with extreme anxiety or psychosis through an unknown mechanism. Lithium is an ion unique among psychoactive drugs in its ability to control mania and some depressions without producing CNS excitation or depression. Its mode of action is unknown. Very recent evidence indicates that calcium channel blocking agents, carbamazepine and propranolol also may have a role in the treatment of some affective disorders.

Indications, contraindications, side effects and interactions with other medications of the recognized somatic therapies for depression are summarized in the table at the end of this chapter.

SELECTION OF AN ANTIDEPRESSANT

Of the available somatic therapies, only tricyclic and tetracyclic antidepressants, and occasionally phenothiazines, are used in the routine office treatment of depression by the primary physician.

Four groups of tricyclics are available:

1. Imipramine (Tofranil) and its demethylated derivatives (e.g., desipramine)

2. Amitriptyline (Elavil) and its demethylated derivatives (e.g., nortriptyline, protriptyline)

3. Doxepin (Sinequan)

4. Amoxapine (Asendin)

Recently, maprotiline (Ludiomil), a tetracyclic antidepressant, has been introduced in the United States. It is about as effective as the tricyclics. Claims that its onset of action is more rapid have not been convincingly substantiated.

The following general guidelines help in choosing between classes of antidepressants:

1. Because amitriptyline and doxepin are more sedating than imipramine, they often are used for depression with anxiety or insomnia

2. The usual daily doses of doxepin and protriptyline are lower than those of imipramine or amitriptyline

3. All antidepressants are dangerous in the immediate post-M.I. period

4. Doxepin and amoxapine may be less cardiotoxic than other antidepressants

5. Protriptyline, amoxapine and maprotiline are less anticholinergic than other preparations

6. Amoxapine seems to have a more rapid onset of action

7. Patients with a past history of a good response to a particular tricyclic should receive that drug again

8. Patients with a family history of a good response to a particular tricyclic can be tried first on that drug

9. If a particular antidepressant is ineffective, the next drug tried should belong to a different class (e.g., switch from amitriptyline to imipramine)

HOW TO PRESCRIBE ANTIDEPRESSANTS

Once a particular tricyclic has been selected, the following guidelines for prescribing it in outpatient practice may be followed:

1. Give the patient one 25 mg. pill of imipramine or amitriptyline or its equivalent to take at bedtime, and have the patient call the next day. If he reports that the drug made him feel terrible, he will be unlikely to take it regularly, and a medication in another class of antidepressant should be prescribed.

2. If the patient tolerates the "test dose" well, increase the dose by 25-50 mg. every other day until a daily dose of 150-200 mg. of imipramine or its equivalent is reached. This may be prescribed initially in divided dosage or as one bedtime dose.

3. Older patients should start at a lower dose, and the final total daily dose should be lower.

4. Once the patient is taking a therapeutic dose of an antidepressant, the total daily dose may be taken at night for several reasons:

   -Anticholinergic side effects are less bothersome when the patient is asleep

   -There are fewer doses to forget

   -Nighttime sedation obviates the need for a sleeping pill

   -Bothersome daytime sedation is minimized

5. Remind the patient that it may take 1-4 weeks at a therapeutic dose before a response occurs.

6. If the patient fails to respond within a month, consider these common causes for the lack of response:

   -The patient may not be taking the drug

   -He may be taking another drug (e.g., a barbiturate) which lowers the blood level of the antidepressant

   -He may need more of the drug to achieve an adequate blood level (up to 250-300 mg. of imipramine or its equivalent may be required)

   -He may be a nonresponder to that particular drug

   -The diagnosis may be in error

7. If the patient complains of anticholinergic side effects (e.g., dry mouth, blurred vision) reassure him that most people develop tolerance to these symptoms. It may also help to tell the patient that the symptoms indicate that the drug is starting to work.

8. Overdose with tricyclics is often lethal: The LD_{50} is about a one-week supply. It therefore makes sense to write prescriptions for no more than a few days' supply of medication at a time if suicide is a concern. This also ensures that the physician remains in frequent contact with the patient.

9. If medications work, continue them for 6 months,
    and then decrease the dose by 25 mg. a week to
    avoid withdrawal symptoms (e.g., nausea, headache,
    and malaise). If symptoms of depression return,
    resume the drug for another 6 months, and attempt
    to taper again. If symptoms return again, the
    patient may need to be maintained on medication for
    prolonged periods of time.

DRUG TREATMENT OF DEPRESSION WITH ANXIETY

Many depressions are accompanied by anxiety. The decision to treat
the anxiety depends on how much is present and its relationship to
the depression.

1. If the patient's primary symptom is anxiety accompanied
    by mild depression, prescribe an antianxiety drug
    (see page 76). Remember that antianxiety drugs may
    worsen or precipitate depression.

2. If the patient has significant depression with some
    anxiety, give a sedating antidepressant (e.g.,
    amitriptyline or doxepin).

3. When depression and anxiety both are significant,
    start with one of the following:

    -Thiroidazine 40-200 mg/day, or other sedating
     antipsychotic drug in low doses

    -A sedating tricyclic antidepressant

4. Fixed combinations of antianxiety drugs and anti-
    depressants (e.g., Limbitrol) may occasionally be
    useful short-term for some patients.

USE OF LITHIUM

Lithium is effective in the treatment and prophylaxis of mania and
the prophylaxis of some recurrent depressions. Although it usually is
prescribed by the psychiatrist, this substance has recently been used
to treat cluster headaches and neutropenia. Because it is potentially
toxic, especially to brain, kidney, heart, thyroid and parathyroid,
the status of these systems is surveyed before lithium is begun.

Areas of function that should periodically be surveyed in patients
taking lithium are described in the left-hand column below. The
rationale for each test can be found in the right-hand column.

Test	*Rationale*
CBC	Lithium may cause leukocytosis
BUN, creatinine, urinalysis	Lithium is excreted by the kidney. Impaired ability to excrete the ion results in toxicity
Creatinine clearance, 24 hour urine volume, at times GFR	Interstitial fibrosis and glomerular and tubular necrosis have been reported in patients on long-term lithium therapy. Renal function should should be monitored yearly
Serum sodium	Sodium and lithium are handled similarly by the renal tubule. Conditions that cause sodium depletion (e.g., salt restriction, vomiting, excess exercise in hot weather, use of diuretics) result in increased reabsorption of lithium along with sodium, leading to lithium toxicity
Mental Status Exam (see pp	Lithium can worsen OBS and schizophrenia, and subtle OBS may be an early sign of lithium toxicity
EKG and chest x-ray in older patients, or where cardiovascular disease is suspected	Lithium can be cardiotoxic and should be used cautiously in patients with cardiac disease
Serum calcium	Longterm lithium therapy may cause hyper-parathyroidism
Thyroid function tests	Lithium may cause goiter and hypothyroidism in patients with a history of thyroid disease
Urine osmolality	Nephrogenic diabetes insipidus often occurs in lithium-treated patients

When prescribing lithium, follow these guidelines:

1. The usual dose range for chronic treatment is 600-1200 mg/day, which can be given in divided dose or as one daily dose

2. The dose should be adjusted to achieve a blood level of 0.6 - 1.2 mEq/l. Many patients can be maintained successfully at 0.6 - 0.8 mEq/l of lithium

3. Blood levels must be drawn 12 hours after the last dose and <u>before</u> the patient's first daily dose, or the transient rise in lithium level that occurs within an hour of ingesting the drug will make the blood level seem higher than it actually is in the steady state

4. In chronic lithium treatment, blood levels should be drawn monthly, more frequently during hot weather or if the patient develops vomiting or diarrhea, when sodium depletion may cause increased lithium reabsorption and higher blood levels

5. Advise the patient to call immediately and to have a lithium level drawn if he notices signs of lithium toxicity, including nausea and vomiting, diarrhea, lethargy, confusion, ataxia, dysarthria and a course tremor, which progress to muscle twitching, fasciculations and clonic contractions, and later to seizures, delirium, and stupor. Serum lithium usually is above 2.0-2.5 mEq/l but may be lower

6. Avoid diets, especially low sodium diets

7. Avoid fluid restriction

8. Doses and blood levels used to treat acute mania are higher (1000-3000 mg/day in divided dose; blood level 0.8-1.5 mEq/l). The amount required decreases as the attack subsides. This condition should be treated by a psychiatrist

9. Renal damage may be prevented by prescribing the lowest possible dose of lithium and by advising the patient to drink 2-3 liters of fluid each day

10. Indications for lithium are summarized in Table 2.1

DIFFERENTIAL DIAGNOSIS

Depression can be confused with several commonly encountered conditions that are considered below, opposite salient differentiating features from the history or examination.

Psychiatric Diagnosis	*Salient Differentiating Features*
Normal sadness or "blues" is usually due to the vagaries of everyday life	-Symptoms are transient and improve when the external situation changes -Symptoms respond to reassurance -Symptoms are not as pervasive as in depression and do not interfere with ability to function -The "depressive triad" is not present
Grief is a normal, self-limited reaction to the loss of an important person. The sadness, agitation, anorexia, and insomnia accompanying grief may be confused with vegetative signs of depression	-Guilt is limited to thoughts about what the patient could have done to save the deceased or to guilt at having survived -Symptoms usually are better in the morning and worse as the day goes on -Acute symptoms subside in 4-6 weeks -Lowered self-esteem is not pronounced in grief -A sense of resolution of sadness occurs in normal grief but not in depression
Organic brain syndrome often presents with depressive symptoms as a reaction to the primary cognitive impairment. Some depressed patients complain of difficulty concentrating, and severely depressed patients may be found to have a mild memory and concentration disturbance on mental status testing (depressive pseudo-dementia) that mimics OBS	-Vegetative signs are absent in OBS -Many depressed patients with "memory trouble" do not have signs of OBS on careful MSE testing in which the patient is encouraged to try his hardest, while MSE is abnormal in OBS with depressive symptoms -The findings on MSE of many patients with "depressive pseudodementia" are not as profound as would be expected from a severe OBS causing severe depression -Careful testing may be required to differentiate depression and OBS -Antidepressants worsen depression due to OBS but improve primary depression

Psychiatric Diagnosis	*Salient Differentiating Features*
Hypochondriasis can be confused with depression accompanied by multiple somatic complaints, especially when the patient does not admit to feeling depressed	-Few vegetative signs are present -Multiple contact with doctors occurs -The depressed patient is more likely to "give up" after an unrewarding contact with a doctor, while hypochondriacs demonstrate illness claiming behavior -A lifelong pattern of complaining exists -There is no history of a recent loss
Schizophrenia's "blunted" or "flat" affect may sometimes be confused with depressive affect, and patients with severe (psychotic) depression may have delusions. Also, schizophrenic patients may experience depression during the course of their illness or after they recover	-The patient feels "empty" rather than sad -Vegetative signs are not present -Disordered thinking, with loose associations, autistic logic, and bizarre and idiosyncratic thinking are present -Delusions in psychotic depression are of guilt or bodily decay -First rank symptoms are absent in depression -The schizophrenic patient does not profound sadness and is unlikely to elicit empathic sadness in the examiner
Medical illnesses can present with depression, even before the condition manifests itself in other ways	Illnesses commonly associated with depression include: -Viral infection (e.g., hepatitis, infectious mononucleosis) -Other infections (e.g., pneumonia) -Tumors (e.g., pancreatic carcinoma) -Endocrine disease (thyroid, adrenal, pituitary and parathyroid) -Multiple sclerosis -Rheumatoid arthritis -Hypokalemia -Anemia, especially pernicious anemia -Systemic lupus erythematosis -Cardiovascular and cerebrovascular disease
Medications and nonprescription drugs may produce depression, especially in patients with a past history of depression	Drugs that commonly produce or aggravate depression include: -Antihypertensives(especially reserpine, alphamethyldopa and spironolactone) -Propranolol -Antianxiety drugs -Oral contraceptives -Adrenal steroids and ACTH -Withdrawal from amphetamines and cocaine -L-dopa -Alcohol

USE OF THE PSYCHIATRIST

The primary physician should <u>consult with the psychiatrist</u>:

1. Whenever suicide is a possibility

2. For help with differential diagnosis

3. For help with psychotherapy planning

4. To understand the psychodynamics of the patient's depression

5. If the patient has had a severe depression in the past

6. If the treatment plan is not working

The primary physician should <u>refer the patient to a psychiatrist</u> if:

1. The patient is clearly suicidal

2. The patient is psychotic

3. Treatment by the primary physician is unsuccessful

4. The patient has an additional severe psychiatric disease (e.g., schizophrenia)

5. The patient wishes longterm psychotherapy for a deeply ingrained personality problem that causes recurrent or chronic depression

6. The physician does not wish to treat the patient's depression

Table 2.1

CHARACTERISTICS OF SOMATIC THERAPIES OF DEPRESSION

Mode of Therapy	Indications	Contra-indications/ Precautions	Some Side Effects	Drug Interactions	Comments
Tricyclics and tetra-cyclics	-Previous response to these classes -Family history of response to a tricyclic or tetracyclic -Panic attacks and some phobias	-Glaucoma -Prostatic hyper-trophy -Use with caution in the presence of a recent M.I., heart block, or congestive heart failure	-Anticholinergic (dry mouth, blurred vision, urinary reten-tion, OBS) -Postural hypo-tension -Precipitation of mania in patients with bi-polar ill-ness (manic de-pressive disease) -Cardiac arrhyth-mia (rare) -Quinidine-like effect	-Interference with the action of antihyperten-sives, especial-ly quanethidine, clonidine and bethanedine -Severe hyperten-sion when given with amphetamines, epinephrine, norepenephorine, phenylephrine and MAO inhibi-tors -Barbiturates and alcohol stimulate meta-bolizing enzymes and decrease blood levels of tricyclics -Decreased effect of L-dopa -Increased pheny-toin toxicity	-Doxepin and amoxapine are safer for patients with heart disease

Table 2.1 Contd.

Mode of Therapy	Indications	Contra-indications/Precautions	Some Side Effects	Drug Interactions	Comments
MAO inhibitors	-Failure to respond to a tricyclic antidepressant -Some atypical depression -Some phobias and panic attacks	-Patient's eating of foods containing tyramine -Heart disease -Unreliable patient	-Hypertension -Irritability -Anorexia -Impotence -Anticholinergic side effects	-Dangerous hypertensive reactions when given with many foods, cyclamates, tricyclic antidepressants, pressor amines, L-dopa, meperidine, and many others	-Should only be prescribed by a psychiatrist familiar with their use
EST	-Severe depression -Imminent suicide risk -When drug therapy is contraindicated -Failure to respond to medication	-Intracranial mass -Increased intracranial pressure	-Confusion and memory loss lasting hours to months -Bradycardia due to vagal stimulation	-CNS toxicity may occur in patients taking lithium who receive ECT	-A safe, extremely effective treatment when administered with an anesthesiologist present -General anesthesia (usually a short-acting barbiturate) plus a muscle relaxant such as succinylcholine eliminate the fear and dis-

Table 2.1 contd.

Mode of Therapy	Indications	Contra-indications/Precautions	Some Side Effects	Drug Interactions	Comments
EST					comfort which used to be associated with this procedure -Unilateral electrodes produce less memory loss
Pheno-thiazines	-Depression with psychosis or severe anxiety	-Glaucoma -Prostatic hypertrophy	-Anticholinergic -Postural hypotension -Parkinsonia symptoms -Cardiac rhythm disturbances	-May interfere with action of antihypertensives -Additive anticholinergic side effects with tricyclics	-Thioridazine (Mellaril) is the most commonly used phenothiazine in the treatment of depression with anxiety -Thioridazine should not be prescribed in doses of more than 800 mg/day

Table 2.1 contd.

Mode of Therapy	Indications	Contra-indications/ Precautions	Some Side Effects	Drug Interactions	Comments
Lithium	-Treatment of acute mania (alone or in combination with an anti-psychotic drug) -Prevention of recurrent attacks of mania -Prevention of recurrent depression when there is a past history of mania (bipolar depression) -Prevention of some recurrent unipolar depressions -Management of cluster headaches and neutropenia	-Severe renal disease -Use with caution in patients with cardiovascular and brain disease	Dose related: -GI symptoms: nausea and vomiting, diarrhea, abdominal pain -Fine tremor -Sleepiness -Dazed feeling -Polyuria and polydipsia Not dose related: -Thyroid enlargement -Nephrogenic diabetes insipidus-like syndrome -Acute OBS -EKG changes -Leukocytosis -Irreversible kidney damage (may be dose related)	-Sodium wasting diuretics result in increased lithium reab-sorption and toxicity -High doses of haloperidol should be used with caution in patients taking lithium -Lithium toxicity may appear when coadministered with antibiotics (especially tetracycline) -Indomethacin and methyldopa increase lithium levels -Phenothiazines may decrease lithium levels	-A potentially lethal sub-stance which should not be prescribed unless blood levels are monitored regularly and the patient is reliable and not acutely suicidal

REFERENCES

Carroll BJ, Feinberg M, Greden JF: A specific laboratory test for the diagnosis of melancholia. Arch Gen Psychiatry 1981; 38:15

Dubovsky SL: Psychotherapeutics in Primary Care New York, Grune and Stratton, 1981. pp 85-114

Havens L: Anatomy of a suicide. N Engl J Med 1965; 272:401

Klerman GJ: Overview of affective disorders. In: Kaplan, et al: Comprehensive Textbook of Psychiatry /III. Baltimore Williams and Wilkins, 1980. pp 1305-1319.

Liberman RP, Raskin DE: Depression: A behavioral formulation. Arch Gen Psychiatry 1971; 24:515

Murphy GL: The physician's responsibility for suicide. Ann Int Med 1975; 82:301, 305.

Ross M: The practical recognition of depressive and suicidal states. Ann Int Med 1966; 64:1079.

Seligman MEP.: Depression and learned helplessness. In: RJ Freedman and M Katz (Eds): The Psychology of Depression. pp 83-125.

Shopsin B, Waters B: The pharmacotherapy of major depressive syndromes. Psychosomatics 1980; 21:542

Chapter Three
ANXIETY

No physician can remain in practice for long without encountering anxious patients. Anxiety is a prominent complaint in 10-15% of medical outpatients and 10% of medical inpatients. In addition, many maladaptive reactions to illness represent attempts to deal with excessive worries about being sick. Even 2-5% of healthy people are incapacitated by anxiety at some time in their lives and some form of anxiety is found in 75% of the normal population. Although an optimal amount of anxiety can be a very adaptive motivating force, too much or inappropriate anxiety can interfere with normal functioning.

Because it represents a psychological response to a real or imagined danger, anxiety is accompanied by the body's mobilization to fight or escape. Symptoms of physiologic arousal that are particularly likely to be prominent in anxious patients include cardiovascular complaints (e.g., tachycardia, palpitations, chest pain), respiratory symptoms (e.g., dyspnea, tachypnea), gastrointestinal distress, musculoskeletal symptoms and general complaints of weakness, diaphoresis, dry mouth and faintness. Excess catecholamine secretion may produce tachyarrhythmias and congestive heart failure in patients with damaged myocardiums.

When acute, anxiety may be accompanied by the hyperventilation syndrome, a state in which hyperventilation and shortness of breath predominate. Fearful that he is not getting enough air, the anxious patient's natural tendency to hyperventilate is increased. The respiratory alkalosis that can result from just 5 deep breaths alters levels of ionized calcium and cerebral blood flow, causing cerebral hypoxia, numbness, parasthesias, lightheadedness and rarely, tetany and loss of consciousness. The patient may not be aware that he is breathing too rapidly. Rebreathing into a paper bag or decreasing one's respiratory rate reverses these changes, while voluntary over-breathing reproduces them.

Many anxious patients with resulting autonomic arousal are aware of their inner tension, although they may assume that their physical symptoms are the cause, rather than the result, of their emotional distress. Other patients, because their somatic symptoms are so prominent that they occupy all of their attention or because they find it difficult to tolerate an awareness of their emotions, are relatively unaware of their underlying anxiety and are convinced that their problem is purely physical. The physician, too, may be unaware that these patients' complaints are due to anxiety until a complete workup reveals no pathology or until he becomes anxious himself in response to the patient's hidden discomfort.

CLUES TO THE DIAGNOSIS OF ANXIETY

Many anxious patients do not realize that feeling ill, out of sorts or in distress is caused by anxiety. The following signs and symptoms may indicate an underlying anxiety disorder:

Physical Clues:

1. Fidgeting and hyperactivity

2. Facial expressions of panic

3. Tachycardia, palpitations, chest pain

4. Shortness of breath, tachypnea

5. Lightheadedness, dizziness

6. Headache

7. Diarrhea, heartburn, abdominal pain

8. Urinary frequency

9. Trembling, faintness

10. Diaphoresis

11. Dry mouth

12. Paresthesias

Psychological Clues:

1. Complaints of tension, worry, fear or nervousness

2. A sense of doom or panic

3. Difficulty concentrating

4. Preoccupation with oneself

5. Complaints of chronic fatigue and lack of energy

6. Feelings that the world seems odd or unreal
    (de-realization) or that the patient is not the same person
    (de-personalization)

7. Problems with sexual performance

8. Abuse of medications or alcohol

9. Accident proneness

ENCOUNTER WITH A TYPICAL PATIENT

Ms. T. is a 38 year-old, divorced nurse who noted a small
lump in her breast a few months ago. She immediately consulted her
physician, and a few weeks later she underwent a mastectomy for
carcinoma. Although her recovery was uneventful, she has continued
to experience pain in the incision and to complain of intermittent
gastrointestinal and respiratory symptoms. Having completed a thorough
workup, her physician relates his findings:

Dr: I've gone over the pathology slides and I'm pleased
     to say that I think we got all the cancer.

Pt: Why do you think the incision still hurts? Shouldn't
     it have healed by now?

Dr: The wound has healed, and we'll soon be able to start
     the restructive surgery we discussed.

Pt: Are you sure that the lymph node resection shouldn't have
     been more extensive? After all, this lightheadedness I've
     been experiencing could be due to brain metastases,
     couldn't it?

Dr: That might be remotely possible, but I really don't think
     it's likely.

Pt: Are you sure? My heart rate has been high - don't you think I
     could have suffered a cardiac complication during surgery?

Dr: I really don't. I think we should consider some other
     explanation for all these symptoms.

Pt: I'm trying not to worry, but I've been reading up on
this and I'm becoming convinced that the cancer could
still be there. How sure are you that it isn't?

THE PHYSICIAN'S REACTION TO HIS PATIENT

Even the apparently calm patient may communicate his underlying
anxiety by subtly inducing a state of inner tension in the doctor
through worried looks, nervous, pressured speech or by covert assaults
on the clinician's confidence. Reactions that are commonly induced by
anxious patients are described in the left-hand column below, while
the meaning of the doctor's reaction is discussed in the right-hand
column.

Physician's Reaction	*Comment*
Becoming unaccountably nervous	Without being aware of it, the physician may respond empathically to the patient's overt or hidden anxiety by becoming anxious himself. The doctor's discomfort may then be the first clue that the patient is anxious
Feeling that the patient has no reason to worry	The clinician who is upset by the patient's anxiety may attempt to minimize it by insisting that the patient's fears are unrealistic
Conviction that the patient's anxiety is entirely justified	Most illnesses are anxiety-provoking. However, the patient who becomes excessively anxious usually is responding to some inner fear related to the specific meaning of the illness to the patient. The physician may focus on reality factors to avoid the more irrational inner significance of the patient's anxiety
Absence of any feelings about an obviously anxious patient	Throughout their medical training, physicians learn to protect themselves emotionally by isolating themselves to some degree from their patients' worries. When a patient is very anxious, the need for this protective mechanism may

be so great that all awareness of the
physician's emotional response to
the patient is avoided

COMMON UNSUCCESSFUL APPROACHES

When anxiety is excessive, it usually represents a response not
only to the real, external environment, but also to fears that have
been stimulated by inner, less realistic ideas. Approaches that
usually are unsuccessful in dealing with this situation are described
below, along with the patient's response and the reasons why this
response occurs.

Physician's Approach	Patient's Response	Explanation
Reassure the patient that his fears are unfounded	After feeling better, the patient's fears increase	Although the patient initially is reassured by the physician's confidence, he soon becomes worried that the doctor does not truly understand the depth of his concerns and does not take him seriously
Agree with the patient that he would be less nervous if people would stop bothering him	Although the patient says that he is pleased that the physician understands him, he continues to complain about the ways in which other people are making him anxious	In blaming others for his distress, the patient avoids recognizing his inner fears and does not accept responsibility for his own contribution to his problems. Since he does not acknowledge an internal problem, he is unable to change it
Perform an extensive workup to rule out all possible organic causes of anxiety	The patient becomes convinced that he is suffering from a serious physical illness	Although a careful medical evaluation is important, excessive focus on unlikely illnesses not only avoids

Physician's Approach	*Patient's Response*	*Explanation*
		recognition of crucial psychological factors, but provides the patient with even more to worry about
Tell the patient that the physician would also be anxious under similar circumstances	The patient's anxiety rapidly increases	The patient feels that if the physician is frightened by the situation, he has even more reason to worry
Prescribe a month's supply of an anti-anxiety drug immediately	The patient calls a week later complaining that he has run out of medication and would like a refill of his prescription	Since the cause of the patient's anxiety has not yet been uncovered, it is impossible to know whether anti-anxiety drugs should be prescribed. Because the patient does not understand his fears, he begins to rely excessively on medication as the only means of controlling them

A SUCCESSFUL APPROACH

If the physician understands why the patient is anxious, he is in a better position to devise a treatment plan and to offer reassurance that is more exactly directed at the patient's worries:

Dr: You seem to be very worried about having metastatic cancer.

Pt: Wouldn't you be worried? How am I supposed to be calm when I've just had a breast removed for cancer?

Dr: It's true that most people would be upset by having had a breast removed; but everyone is different, and people have different specific concerns.

Pt: Well, I'm 38 years old and I've been so involved in my career that I haven't thought about getting remarried.

Now I'm ~~worried that my time is limited and I'll~~
never find anyone to share my life with.

Dr: This sounds like an issue that was important even
       before the cancer.

Pt: Yes, but it's much worse now. I've always prided myself
       on being attractive and...

Dr: Go on...

Pt: I'm afraid that if I talk about these things, they
       may come true.

Dr: You may find that putting your fears into words
       actually makes them easier to handle.

Pt: If you think so, I'll try. Well, I have been feeling
       that I'll never be the same again, and that now I'll
       never be able to accomplish what I wanted to in life.
       But I've always been an independent person and I don't
       want to bother you with all this.

Dr: The more you keep your worries to yourself, the harder
       it is to find ways to overcome them. If we put our heads
       together, I think that we can learn a little more about
       why these concerns are so strong for you and then find
       ways of dealing more effectively with them.

An attitude of realistic confidence in the physician's ability
to understand the patient's anxiety, to offer support, and at least
to find ways of controlling the patient's symptoms can be enormously
reassuring to the patient who feels temporarily overwhelmed by fears
that he does not entirely understand. The physician may then proceed
with the following general measures:

1. Rule out organic illnesses and medications that may present
    with anxiety. Some diseases cause anxiety by stimulating
    the sympathetic nervous system or producing tachycardia,
    while others' mechanism of action in producing this symptom
    is unclear. Conditions and drugs to consider are listed
    on page 72

2. Clarify with the patient what in the present situation is so
    frightening. As the patient begins a search for the meaning
    of his anxiety, he begins to gain a sense of control over it.

3. Determine the patient's capacity for self-awareness. Some

patients are interested in learning more about hidden psychological factors that are making them anxious. When these
patients know more about the reasons for their anxiety, they
are able to find more adaptive solutions to their problems.
However, forcing insight on patients who do not wish to look
into themselves is likely to be experienced as a threat and
to increase anxiety.

4. <u>Support existing coping abilities and assess techniques that
   have worked in the past.</u> Asking the patient about ways in
   which he has reacted to stress in the past often reveals
   characteristic ways of coping with anxiety. When a particular
   approach has proved successful, it is likely to work again
   when anxiety recurs. For example, the patient who went back
   to work soon after a myocardial infarction in the past can be
   encouraged to become active as quickly as medically feasible
   if he becomes frightened by a recent heart attack. Some
   patients use intellectual defenses. Therefore, these people
   do better when they are given full information about their
   illnesses and care.

5. <u>Give the patient as much control over his care as feasible.</u>
   Because the anxious patient feels helpless and overwhelmed,
   any maneuver that increases his sense of mastery over the
   situation is likely to be reassuring. While anxiety will
   increase if the patient is given a task he cannot handle, the
   physician should not do anything for the patient that he cannot
   do for himself.

6. <u>Offer ongoing support when the patient's strengths are limited.</u>
   Many patients, for example, those with chronic organic brain
   syndromes (dementias) and some personality disorders, are
   limited in their ability to cope with life's stresses and
   become anxious in response even to minor setbacks. These
   patients require ongoing advice, support and assistance in
   mobilizing necessary resources from family members, friends
   and social agencies, and help in achieving realistic expectations. Regular ongoing appointments with the physician
   should be increased at times of stress.

7. <u>Consider adjunctive techniques when they are suited to the
   patient's personality and the physician's preferences.</u>
   Relaxation, meditation and hypnosis can be useful techniques
   for patients who are able to relax under the direction of an
   authority figure, while biofeedback can be prescribed for
   patients who need a visual or auditory signal to assess their
   level of tension. Systematic desensitization, a technique
   usually applied by a specialist, involves teaching the patient
   to relax and then encouraging him to think about progressively
   more anxiety-provoking situations. When frightening thoughts

are paired with relaxation, they gradually lose their ability
to evoke anxiety and the patient eventually is able to face
calmly situations that used to make him anxious.

APPROACH TO SPECIFIC TYPES OF ANXIETY
MEDICAL PATIENTS MAY EXPERIENCE

Like pain, anxiety is a nonspecific response to inner distress
whose cause must be elucidated before it is treated. Once the physician
has gained the patient's confidence, he is in a position to determine
why the patient is anxious and then to apply specific techniques aimed
at the underlying cause of the patient's distress. Often it is not
clear what sort of anxiety the patient is experiencing; frequently,
the causes may be mixed. For example, a patient who is fearful of
dependency also may be frightened of dying. In addition, techniques
useful for one type of anxiety also are useful in other situations.
Categories of anxiety experienced by medical patients are described in
the left-hand column below, while the right-hand column outlines an
approach to management.

Category of Anxiety	*Therapeutic Approach*
Situational Anxiety. Severe stress may temporarily overwhelm anyone's coping abilities and produce severe anxiety that usually abates as the situation resolves. Because even a clear external danger may remind the patient of previously unresolved inner conflicts, situational anxiety may be accompanied by any of the other types of anxiety described below.	-Reduce anxiety rapidly through reassurance, suggestion, emotional support, medication and adjunctive techniqeus (e.g., hypnosis) -Where feasible, attempt to modify anxiety-provoking situations -Avoid attempts at providing insight into long-standing conflicts in acutely anxious patients -Clarify with the patient exactly what about the present situation is so frightening
Anxiety about bodily damage or loss of prowess or attractiveness. While most patients worry about the effects on their appearance of surgery or illnesses that may be mutilating, individuals who feel that love and approval from others are only forthcoming if they are physically attractive may be especially threatened. These	-Without being dishonest, attempt to find traits that indicate that the patient still is attractive or strong -Remind the patient of the positive physical attributes that remain -Acknowledge the patient's efforts to assert his strength, For example, praise his courage in cooperating with a treatment plan

Category of Anxiety	*Therapeutic Approach*

patients may become convinced that minor abnormalities or complications indicate that they are permanently damaged or they may attempt to reassure themselves by demonstrating their attractiveness or strength in inappropriate ways, e.g., by behaving seductively, or exercising conspicuously in dangerous ways (e.g., soon after a myocardial infarction)

that requires him to rest when he feels strong and healthy
-Assess the impact of a change in appearance on the patient's spouse
-Realistically discuss what the patient can do to replace lost function (e.g., mammoplasty)
-Encourage mourning of lost beauty or function

Fear of death. Even nonfatal illnesses can remind a patient of his mortality. However, because it is difficult to think of oneself as being dead, a preoccupation with the prospect of dying often symbolizes other concerns, such as fear of pain, isolation, helplessness, and the impending loss of important relationships

-Encourage the patient to discuss all of his feelings about the meaning of death
-Evaluate emotional or physical withdrawal of significant people in the patient's life
-Reassure the patient that pain will be treated adequately
-Promise ongoing understanding and support
-Prevent isolation of the patient from nursing staff and physicians

Anxiety about loss of self-esteem. Patients with a fragile sense of self-worth may attempt to bolster their self-esteem through protestations of their importance. These individuals become anxious if an illness is perceived as a personal failure or as an imperfection. They may attempt to enhance their self-image by treating the physician as an unworthy subordinate or by insisting that they associate only with the most prestigious physicians

-Avoid the temptation to retaliate by proving to the patient that he is not as special as he thinks
-Maintain an appropriately deferential attitude
-Attempt to find something admirable about the patient
-Provide special considerations that do not interfere with medical care
-Allow the patient to express admiration for the primary physician, a senior colleague, or a consultant

Separation anxiety. Hospitalized patients, particularly those who are regressed (see pp. 165-168) may, like small children, become

-Allow unrestricted visiting, especially during procedures and at night
-Provide a nightlight

Category of Anxiety

Therapeutic Approach

frightened when they are separated
from important and familiar
people. Somatic complaints,
demands for attention (e.g.,
repeatedly ringing for the nurse)
more direct expressions of anxiety
and fears that caretakers will not
return, appear when the patient is
left alone, even for a few minutes

-Ask family members to provide
  familiar objects for the patient's
  room
-Have nursing staff and other
  personnel visit the patient
  frequently for brief periods of
  time. Longer visits at greater
  intervals are less likely to reduce
  the patient's complaints than are
  brief but frequent interactions
  that are not contingent on the
  patient's repeatedly asking for
  company
-Attempt to provide consistent
  coverage by the same nurses each
  day
-Reassure the patient that the
  treatment relationship will be
  consistent and that the patient
  will not be deserted by health-
  care providers

Stranger anxiety. Signs of distress may appear when children
and regressed adults are confronted
by new caretakers (e.g., new house
officers), especially if separation
anxiety also is present

-Minimize cross-coverage
-When possible, introduce the
  patient to new physicians and
  nurses before he must begin working
  with them, e.g., during vacations
  or when house officers change
  service
-Provide additional support from
  familiar personnel while the
  patient is becoming accustomed to
  new major caretakers

Fear of loss of control. When
they become ill, patients with a
strong need to be self-sufficient
may feel that they are no longer
in control of their own lives
because others must make important
decisions for them (e.g., about
which medications, when to eat, or
when to get out of bed). They may
then attempt to assert some control
over the physician by complaining
about their care, refusing to
take medications as prescribed
or to acknowledge improvement,

-Allow as many choices as possible
  about treatment, e.g., by asking
  the patient when it would be best
  for him to take medications or
  whether he thinks a particular
  test seems reasonable
-Provide opportunities for the
  patient to question the diagnosis
  and treatment plan
-Avoid power struggles in which
  the physician attempts to control
  the patient by refusing to
  accede to reasonable demands
-Within the limits of good medical

Category of Anxiety   *Therapeutic Approach*

doubting the physician's ability
to help them, and demanding rather
than requesting information and
specific therapies. Fear of loss
of control often accompanies
anxiety about dependency and
closeness

care, allow the outpatient to
determine the date of the next
appointment

Fear of dependency. Some patients
whose normal needs to be cared
for were not met earlier in life
protect themselves from an awareness of strong dependency wishes
that feel overpowering by insisting
on their autonomy and self-
sufficiency. These individuals
feel threatened when an illness,
temporary disability, aging, or the
development of a close relationship threatens their hyperindependent stance. Hostility
toward those on whom the patient
is tempted to depend, complaints
about how dependent others are on
him, and efforts to reject others'
efforts to be helpful, e.g.,
through noncompliance and failure
to keep appointments, represent
attempts by the patient to prove
to himself that he does not need
to rely on anyone

-Reassure the acutely ill patient
 that his state of dependency is
 only temporary
-Allow the patient to complain
 about his care
-Convey an understanding of the
 patient's discomfort at being
 cared for
-Discharge the patient as rapidly
 as possible
-Avoid excessive kindness and
 solicitousness that may stimulate
 underlying dependency wishes
-Allow the patient to determine the
 frequency of appointments with the
 physician
-Involve the patient in treatment
 planning as much as possible
-Help the patient with a chronic
 illness to remain as independent
 as possible
-Point out that it is possible to
 depend on others for medical care
 while retaining independence in
 other areas
-When anxiety about depending on a
 spouse is present, consider in-
 volving the partner in treatment

Fear of closeness. Patients who
prefer to maintain their distance
from other people may be particularly threatened by the intense
interactions that are common on
a hospital ward or when a partner
in a relationship suddenly
demands more closeness. The more
other people express interest and
concern, the more anxious these
patients become

-Avoid forcing intimacy on the
 patient
-Maintain a professional demeanor
-Uncover reasons why the partner
 wants to be closer to the patient
 and help him or her to regain
 the previous interpersonal
 distance

Category of Anxiety	*Therapeutic Approach*
"Confessional anxiety". What seems to be nonspecific anxiety actually may represent fear of being ridiculed, shamed or thought of as abnormal or crazy if the patient discusses sexual problems, disturbing thoughts or other embarrassing concerns. Adolescents may be especially worried about discussing masturbation, premarital sex or a desire for contraceptives	-Maintain a nonjudgmental attitude -If the source of the patient's anxiety is not clear, ask if he has any concerns that feel embarrassing or uncomfortable -Help the patient to state concerns openly by putting them into words for him, e.g., by saying, "Do you mean that you think you might be pregnant?"
Anxiety due to the anticipation of punishment. Patients with an underlying sense of guilt about a real or imagined transgression, or those who were never wanted by their parents and who feel that they do not deserve to be happy or even to be alive, often expect, consciously or unconsciously, to be found out and punished. If punishment is not forthcoming, e.g., in the form of an illness that the patient considers just desserts for his sins, the patient may bring it on himself rather than wait passively for the inevitable. Chronically unhappy marriages, accident proneness, failure to improve medically, alcoholism, suicide or unhappiness at work all may serve to ensure that the patient never is happy for too long and that he receives ongoing punishment	-Discuss the patient's guilt feelings openly -Uncover the reasons why the patient feels so guilty -Remain alert for multiple forms of self-destructive behavior -Empathize with the suffering that the patient has experienced in life
Signal anxiety. When a psychological conflict of which the patient is unaware arises for the first time or when a conflict that has remained dormant is stimulated by some event (e.g., the patient's age recalls the age of an important figure in the past), anxiety may arise that signals that psychological equilibrium has been upset	-Attempt to discern the nature of the underlying conflict -Obtain psychiatric consultation to determine which treatment approach to apply

Category of Anxiety	*Therapeutic Approach*
Anxiety may be free-floating, or it may be accompanied by manifestations of defenses against anxiety such as obsessions or phobias	
Anxiety about the emergence of another emotion. When the patient is particularly vulnerable to an emotional state (often depression), he may conceal it from himself, becoming anxious whenever it threatens to emerge	-Identify the underlying affect -Direct treatment at the hidden state (e.g., prescribe an antidepressant if depression is suspected) -Assess the patient's ability, with the doctor's support, to tolerate an awareness of the disguised emotion
Psychotic anxiety. Early psychotic disorganization due to OBS, schizophrenia, mania or borderline states often produces diffuse anxiety as the patient loses control of mental processes	-Perform a thorough mental status exam (see pp. 86-91) -Convey an appreciation of the patient's fear of psychic disorganization -Treat the underlying condition

APPROACH TO MEDICATION

During the past few years, physicians and the public have become increasingly concerned about the growing use of antianxiety drugs in the United States (diazepam still is prescribed more frequently than any other drug). When tranquilizers are given in place of understanding, support and interpersonal therapies, especially to patients who are at risk of abusing medications, this concern is justified, since the patient is taught to rely on a pill rather than on his inner resources to solve his problems. However, recent evidence indicates that when antianxiety drugs are used to facilitate the therapeutic effects of the doctor-patient relationship, they are not misused by the majority of medical patients.

Several classes of antianxiety and other drugs, described in detail on pp. 76-8, are used to reduce anxiety. The following are useful guidelines when prescribing these medications for anxiety or insomnia:

1. Consider using antianxiety agents when anxiety appears acutely in response to an external stress, in a patient

who is motivated to improve and cooperates with treatment.

2. Avoid barbiturates and meprobamate, which may produce
    addiction and dangerous abstinence syndromes and are
    lethal when taken in overdose. Benzodiazepines are safer
    (although they too can be abused) and often are more
    effective than antihistamines and propranolol.

3. Under ordinary circumstances, do not prescribe benzo-
    diazepines for more than 2-4 weeks. However, some
    patients with unremitting situational problems or severe
    personality weaknesses may need long-term drug therapy.

4. Avoid long-term drug therapy of insomnia. Tryptophane,
    benzodiazepines (especially flurazepam and temazepam),
    and antihistamines are much safer than barbiturates and
    related drugs. Sleep disturbances caused by
    depression usually respond to antidepressants and do not
    require an additional drug.

5. If the patient does not improve within a week of
    beginning medication, he is unlikely to benefit from
    that drug and it should be changed or discontinued.

6. Prescribe adequate doses. If insufficient amounts are
    prescribed because of fear of producing addiction, the
    patient is likely to become preoccupied with his symptom,
    and with the drug, when his anxiety is not relieved.

7. Prescribe benzodiazepines in one or two daily doses to
    make use of their long half-lives. A single bedtime
    dose may minimize daytime sedation.

8. Avoid prescribing benzodiazepines for more than a week
    or two, if at all, to patients with a history of
    alcoholism or drug abuse. Physical dependence is a
    particular danger in any patient when daily doses of
    40-60 mg. of diazepam, 100-150 mg. of chlordiazepoxide,
    60-90 mg. of chlorazepate or their equivalents are taken
    for more than one month. Dependence and abstinence
    syndromes also have been reported to occur with lower
    doses of these drugs.

9. Warn the patient that many people experience difficulty
    sleeping for a few days after antianxiety medications
    are discontinued. This does not represent re-emergence
    of the patient's anxiety and is not an indication for
    restarting the drug.

10. Use lower doses and shorter-acting preparations (e.g., lorazepam) of all benzodiazepines and antidepressants in the elderly. Since older patients tend to wake up earlier and sleep less during the night, complaints of disturbed sleep may be due to the normal aging process and drug treatment should be avoided. A nap during the day is likely to be as effective unless the patient is unwavering in his insistence on a sleeping pill.

DIFFERENTIAL DIAGNOSIS

A number of psychiatric and medical illnesses can be confused with primary anxiety states. These are described below, along with salient differentiating features.

Psychiatric Diagnosis	*Salient Differentiating Features*
Many <u>medical illnesses</u> may produce anxiety through their effects on the brain, sympathetic nervous system or catecholamine production before any other signs of disease are evident	<u>Tumors</u>: insulinoma, carcinoid, pheochromocytoma <u>Neurologic</u>: Multiple sclerosis, temporal lobe epilepsy, organic brain disease of any etiology, Meniere's disease <u>Endocrine/Metabolic</u>: Hypoglycemia, thyroid disease, parathyroid disease (especially hypocalcemia), Cushing's Syndrome, porphyria <u>Cardiovascular</u>: Mitral valve prolapse, arteriosclerotic heart disease, paroxysmal tachycardias <u>Pulmonary</u>: COPD, pulmonary embolus, asthma, hypoxia <u>Drug related</u>: Withdrawal states, intoxications (especially amphetamines), akathisia, caffeinism, monosodium glutamate - Chinese restaurant syndrome <u>Infectious</u>: Tuberculosis, brucellosis
<u>Schizophrenia</u> occasionally presents with complaints of anxiety as the psychotic process begins to overwhelm the patient's tenuous	-The schizophrenic patient usually admits to having experienced unusual or bizarre thoughts -First-rank symptoms and other

Psychiatric Diagnosis	*Salient Differentiating Features*
efforts to control it. The severity of the underlying disturbance may only be uncovered by a careful examination	schizophrenic findings can be uncovered by careful questioning
Depression frequently is mixed with anxiety. In fact, 20% of patients who are diagnosed as having an anxiety state turn out to have a primary affective disorder	-Affective disorders have their onset later in life (in the late 30's or early 40's) while anxiety states occur earlier -Patients with anxiety states tend to be worse at night; depressives are worse upon awakening -Patients with depression may have a family history of depression, mania, suicide, alcoholism, and antisocial behavior -Depressive triad (e.g., vegetative signs, sense of worthlessness) is present in depression, absent in anxiety states
Phobias are characterized by anxiety and irrational avoidance of certain situations such as being in public places or elevators	-Anxiety is restricted to the situation of which the patient is phobic -The patient's activities are increasingly restricted until avoidance of the feared situation predominates
Panic disorder consists of recurrent, sudden, unpredictable attacks of intense panic lasting minutes to hours. Anxiety in anticipation of having a panic attack may develop. This anticipatory anxiety may respond to behavior therapy or antianxiety drugs, while the panic states may abate with antidepressants	-3 or more unprovoked panic attacks in a 3 week period -Except for anticipatory anxiety, the patient is not anxious when not experiencing a panic attack -In addition to signs of physiologic arousal, the patient may experience fears of losing control or going crazy during the attack

Psychiatric Diagnosis	*Salient Differentiating Features*
The hyperventilation syndrome may be the presenting complaint in anxious patients, who may not be aware that anxiety is causing their symptoms (see p. 57)	-Lightheadedness, paresthesias, weakness and carpopedal spasm predominate -Symptoms abate with reassurance, voluntary decrease of respiratory rate or rebreathing into a paper bag -Symptoms reappear when the patient breathes rapidly and deeply for three minutes -Past history of hyperventilation may be present
Post-traumatic stress reaction (traumatic neurosis) has received recent news coverage as some Viet Nam veterans have developed delayed reactions to the overwhelming stress of battle overseas followed by an ambivalent welcome back to this country. When opportunities are not provided to vent feelings about the trauma, the patient may continue to re-experience the event repetitively with frightening clarity. Symptoms may begin immediately after the traumatic event, or their onset may be delayed by months or years. Traumatic neurosis can follow any obviously traumatic event	-Recurrent intrusive recollections of the trauma -Recurrent dreams related to the trauma -Sudden periods of feeling that the event is happening again -Easy startling -Disturbed sleep -Guilt about having survived, or about what the patient had to do to survive -Avoidance of activities that remind the patient of the event, with an intensification of symptoms when the patient is exposed to them -Poor memory for the traumatic event

USE OF THE PSYCHIATRIST

The primary physician should consult with a psychiatrist when:

1. The reasons why the patient is anxious are not clear

2. The physician is unsure about which treatment approach to apply

3. The patient has a history of dependence on antianxiety drugs or alcohol

4. The patient is psychotic

5. Anxiety did not arise in the context of a relatively clearcut stress

6. The therapeutic approach is not working

7. The physician feels uncomfortable working with the patient

if: The primary physician should <u>refer the patient to a psychiatrist</u>

1. Anxiety is accompanied by multiple neurotic symptoms such as obsessions and phobias

2. The patient has a history of antisocial behavior or severe addiction

3. The patient is poorly motivated to improve

4. The patient requests intensive psychotherapy for a long-standing personality problem that results in his repetitively feeling anxious

5. The patient requires specialized techniques such as insight psychotherapy, hypnosis or systematic desensitization

6. The patient has a post-traumatic stress disorder

7. The patient arouses strong emotions in the primary physician that make it difficult to work effectively with him

8. The physician does not wish to treat the patient's anxiety

Table 3.1

CHARACTERISTICS OF ANTIANXIETY MEDICATIONS

Class	Examples	Usual daily dose, mg.	Side Effects & Interactions	Comments
Benzo-diazepines	-Diazepam (Valium)	10-20	-Additive sedative effects with other CNS depressants	-Probably the safest and most effective tran-quilizers
	-Chlordiazepoxide (Librium)	20-50	-Abstinence syndromes similar to barbiturate abstinence but later in onset and often less severe may occur at any dose, but especially when more than 40-60 mg/day of diazepam or equivalent are taken (see p.138)	-Fears of widespread abuse of these drugs probably are exaggerated
	-Chlorazepate (Tranxene)	15-22.5		-Flurazepam is a safe hypnotic (sleeping pill) that does not disrupt REM sleep. Relief of insomnia may not appear until the second night of treatment
	-Oxazepam (Serax)	30-45		
	-Flurazepam (Dalmane)	15-30	-Cimetidiene increases blood levels of diazepam and chlordiazepoxide	-Temazepam is a new hypnotic with a shorter half-life than flurazepam
	-Temazepam (Restoril)	30		
Sedative-autonomic antihis-tamines	-Hydroxyzine (Atarax)	100-200	-Anticholinergic side effects are additive with other anticholinergic drugs	-Tolerance and dependence do not occur; however, anxiety reduction is less predictable than with benzodiazepines
	-Diphenhydramine (Benadryl)	100-200	-Sedative effects additive with other CNS depress-ants	-Also useful as hypnotics, especially in older patients
			-G.I. distress, CNS disturbances (e.g., vertigo, tinnitus) and allergy to the drug may occur	

Table 3.1

Class	Examples	Usual daily dose, mg.	Side Effects & Interactions	Comments
Beta-blocking agents	-Propranolol (Inderal)	40-120	-May worsen asthma -Slowing of heart rate may cause exercise intolerance -May cause depression in vulnerable individuals	-Particularly useful when autonomic manifestations of anxiety (e.g., tachycardia) are prominent -Useful when addiction is a concern -Not always effective in relieving anxiety
Tricyclic antidepressants	-Imipramine (Tofranil)	50-300	-See p. 52	-Indicated when anxiety is secondary to or conceals depression -Useful in the treatment of panic attacks and some phobias
Monoaminine oxidase inhibitors	-phenelzine	45-90	-Extremely dangerous interactions with many drugs and foods (see p.53)	-Prescribed only by experts experienced in their use -Also may be useful for panic attacks and phobic-anxiety states
Antipsychotic drugs	-Haloperidol (Haldol) -Thioridazine (Mellaril)	1-5 10-100	-See pp. 250-252	-Indicated for psychotic anxiety -Low doses of nonsedating antipsychotic drugs may reduce anxiety in patients who fear sedation

Table 3.1

Class	Examples	Usual daily dose, mg.	Side Effects & Interactions	Comments
Barbiturates and related drugs	-Phenobarbital	15-60	-Barbiturates enhance microsomal enzymes, reducing blood levels of many other drugs -Life-threatening abstinence syndromes may occur on withdrawal -Tolerance, dependence and addiction are not uncommon -Barbiturates, glutethimide and ethchlorvinyl may precipitate acute porphyria in vulnerable patients	-Because of their propensity for producing addiction and their danger when withdrawn or taken in overdose, these drugs should not be prescribed as anti-anxiety drugs or hypnotics unless other means are ineffective or special circumstances prevail
	-Pentobarbital (Nembutal)	100-200		
	-Secobarbital (Seconal)	100-200		
	-Ethchlorvinyl (Placidyl)	500-1000		
	-Glutethimide (Doriden)	250-500		
	-Meprobamate (Miltown)	400-800		

-Anticholinergic side effects may help some patients with gastrointestinal symptoms
-Keep in mind danger of tardive dyskinesia

REFERENCES

Cole JO: The clinical use of antianxiety drugs. In: Bernstein JG (ed): Clinical Psychopharmacology. Littleton, Mass., PSG Publishing, 1978. pp 19-26

Engel GL: Sudden and rapid death during psychological stress: Folk lore or folk wisdom? Ann Intern Med 1973; 74: 771

Hollister LE: Clinical Use of Psychotherapeutic Drugs. Springfield, Ill., C.C. Thomas, 1973

Kahana R, Bibring G: Personality types in medical management. In: Zinberg NE (ed): Psychiatry and Medical Practice in a General Hospital. New York: International Universities Press, 1964. pp 108-123

Linn L: Clinical manifestations of psychiatric disorders. In: Kaplan et al (eds): Comprehensive Textbook of Psychiatry/III. Baltimore, Williams & Wilkins, 1980. pp 990-1034

Nemiah JC: Anxiety states. In: Kaplan et al (eds): Comprehensive Textbook of Psychiatry/III. Baltimore, Williams & Wilkins, 1980. pp 1483-1493

Sheehan DV: Extreme manifestations of anxiety in the general hospital. In: Hackett TP, Cassem NH: Massachusetts General Hospital Handbook of General Hospital Psychiatry. St. Louis, CV Mosby, 1978. pp 141-173

Strain JJ, Grossman S: Psychological Care of the Medically Ill. New York, Appleton, 1975. pp 23-36

Chapter Four

ORGANIC BRAIN SYNDROMES

Organic brain syndromes (OBS) are a group of disorders characterized by alterations in thinking, emotions or behavior resulting from the direct or indirect effects of organic disease on the brain. They are the most common cause of personality change and psychosis in medically ill patients. Understanding these disorders is easier if the physician is familiar with the effects of changes in brain function on consciousness.

Consciousness refers to those functions that permit awareness and the recording of perceptual information. It may be said to be present if alertness, attention, orientation, and memory can be demonstrated. Normal consciousness requires that the cerebral cortex and brainstem activating mechanisms (reticular activating system or RAS) be intact. Diffuse disturbances of cortical structure or metabolism, and/or diffuse or focal lesions in the reticular activating system, can produce disordered consciousness. When the patient is not unconscious, and the disturbance of consciousness is acute, the resulting acute organic brain syndrome (acute OBS or delirium) consists of an acute, global, disturbance of alertness, attention, orientation, and memory, and the emotional and behavioral reactions to this primary disorder of consciousness. Regardless of the underlying condition that causes an OBS, fluctuation is almost invariably a hallmark, with symptoms appearing to clear, often when the patient is with familiar people, only to worsen at night or when the patient is in strange surroundings.

Chronic organic brain syndromes are also referred to as dementias. They demonstrate less fluctuation, and usually are more insidious in onset. Disturbed alertness and attention are less obvious than disordered orientation, memory and intellect, and fluctuation may be less prominent. Anxiety, agitation and other "emergency" psychological reactions to disturbed cognition, although present, often are less obvious than in delirium because the patient has had more time to adapt to his cognitive deficit.

Symptoms of the disturbance of consciousness in organic brain syndromes often are obscured by more obvious "secondary" reactions, which represent an exaggeration of the usual way in which the patient reacts to any emotionally stressful situation and which usually become the patient's presenting complaint. In most cases, more is learned from these reactions about the patient's character than about the cause of abnormal brain function. Common reactions to the primary disorder of consciousness include:

80

1. Emotional disturbances: A combination of the psychological
    impact on the patient of not being able to think straight
    and possibly the direct effects of the illness on the
    limbic system produce a number of changes in affect:

    -Anxiety is an extremely common reaction to a
    sudden disruption in the ability to think in a
    patient who cannot understand what has happened
    to him.

    -Depression also is a frequently encountered response
    to a loss of cognitive ability. In an attempt to
    explain to himself why he is depressed, and in an
    effort to deny his cognitive deficit, he may invoke
    psychosocial factors that at least feel familiar.
    Since most people, especially if they are sick,
    have had depressing experiences, the patient may
    appear to have a primary depression until the
    underlying disorder of consciousness is uncovered.

    -Anger may represent a way of warding off anxiety,
    or the patient's attempt to protect himself from
    imagined danger.

    -Apathy sometimes is mistaken for depression.

    -Many patients exhibit labile, shallow affect:
    emotional expression fluctuates rapidly and,
    while appropriate to the situation, lacks real
    force. For example, a slightly sad story may
    provoke sudden profuse crying with which the
    examiner finds it difficult to empathize and
    which rapidly abates.

2. Behavioral changes: Agitation, belligerence, and
    psychomotor retardation represent behavioral reactions
    to anxiety, anger and depression, respectively.

3. Perceptual distortions: The "organic" patient's
    ability to perceive reality is disrupted by his
    decreased attention span, memory deficit and
    disruption of perceptual pathways. The patient
    then may misperceive his environment and, in a
    confused and often frightened manner, misinterpret
    events in an attempt to explain situations he
    cannot understand. Visual hallucinations are
    common, although any type of hallucination may
    occur. Illusions, which are misperceptions of actual

stimuli, also are common in OBS. Delusions usually
are concerned with real-life events, and often center
around fears of being in danger from physicians or
hospital staff whom the patient mistakes for dangerous
adversaries.

4. Release of underlying psychopathological processes:
As they grow up, people develop characteristic ways
of reducing anxiety, called character or personality
traits. Situations that increase anxiety, e.g.,
the disturbance of consciousness in organic brain
disease, may result in an exaggeration of character
traits in an attempt to contain increased anxiety.
For example, a patient who tends to ruminate excessively
when he is anxious may respond to disordered
consciousness by becoming so obsessional as to
appear to have an obsessional neurosis. When the
patient has an underlying tendency to use psychotic
symptoms under conditions that cause extreme anxiety,
a psychosis (e.g., schizophrenia) may be precipitated
by organic brain disease. At these times, only very
careful cognitive testing will reveal the organic
disorder that has evoked the psychosis.

Organic brain syndromes can be confused with virtually any
psychiatric disorder, from neurosis to psychosis to character disorder.
Diagnosis therefore rests on the demonstration of the underlying
disorder of consciousness. This is accomplished by utilizing the
mental status examination (MSE) and a variety of special tests of
brain function.

CLUES TO THE DIAGNOSIS OF ORGANIC BRAIN SYNDROME (OBS)

1. Sudden onset ("functional" disorders may appear to
have a sudden onset, but the patient usually has
been deteriorating for days to months)

2. Fluctuating symptoms

3. Older patient (younger patients also may develop OBS)

4. Negative past history of psychiatric disorder

5. Onset or worsening at night ("sundowning")

6. Disorientation to time and place

7. Short-term memory disturbance

8. Illusions and visual or tactile hallucinations

9. Absence of obvious psychological precipitants

10. Worsening of symptoms when drugs that depress
    brain function (e.g., barbiturates) are prescribed

ENCOUNTER WITH A TYPICAL PATIENT

Mr. O. is a 50 year-old man admitted to the Coronary Care Unit
after an acute myocardial infarction. He has no past history of
medical or psychiatric illness. During his first few days in the
hospital he is calm and cooperative. At 10:00 p.m. on his third
hospital day, however, his nurse reports that Mr. O. is having
trouble sleeping. When the doctor stops by to see him, Mr. O. appears
a little restless and says that he is worried about his business.
The doctor reassures him and prescribes a sleeping medication.

At 2:00 a.m. there is an urgent call: Mr. O. wants to sign out
of the hospital. When the physician arrives, the patient is attempting to get dressed. When the physician asks what the problem is, the
following interaction occurs:

Pt: Wrong? Nothing's wrong! (Stops, mutters and
    appears distracted--then startles) Who are you anyway?

Dr: I just talked to you a few hours ago--I'm your
    doctor. What's the problem?

Pt: (Distracted, looking around the room) What's that
    on the wall? Who are those other people?
    (Points to I.V. poles).

Dr: That's just an I.V. pole. There isn't anyone
    there. Calm down.

Pt: You want to hurt me. Stay away...you won't get me!
    (Runs toward the door, knocking over his I.V. and
    ripping the ECG leads off his chest).

THE PHYSICIAN'S REACTION TO HIS PATIENT

Because they are confusing and frightening as well as confused and frightened, patients with organic brain syndromes may evoke strong reactions in their physicians. Common feelings are noted below, along with comments about the doctor's response.

Physician's Approach	*Comment*
Conviction that the patient is schizophrenic	Many people equate "crazy" behavior with schizophrenia, and the delusions and hallucinations of the delirious patient may initially seem schizophrenic. However, since less than 1% of the general population (including the medically ill) is schizophrenic, any psychotic patient is statistically more likely to have an organic brain syndrome
Concern that the patient is simulating or neurotic and is trying to "manipulate" the doctor	When the patient is grossly impaired at one time and apparently clear the next, the physician who does not realize that fluctuation is characteristic of symptoms of OBS may feel that the patient is consciously or unconsciously producing his symptoms
Fear of the patient	The physician who empathizes with the delirious patient's loss of control may justifiably feel frightened of the patient's capacity to act violently

COMMON UNSUCCESSFUL APPROACHES

Mr. O. now is so agitated that he must be quieted if he is to be examined further. Common approaches to calming the agitated patient who may have an OBS are listed in the left-hand column below. The patient's response is listed in the middle column, and an explanation for this reaction can be found in the right-hand column.

Physician's Approach	*Patient's Response*	*Explanation*
Tell the patient to control himself	The patient becomes increasingly belligerent	The patient is so confused that he is unable to control himself. When the physician does not provide the necessary external controls, the patient feels increasingly frightened and his attempts to protect himself through aggression increase
Allow the patient to run off the ward, assuming that he will come back when he feels better	The patient leaves the ward and refuses to return	The patient's loss of control is frightening to him. If the doctor does not take control, the patient's fear of losing control increases. He then attempts to leave the setting in which he is frightened
Without assistance, attempt to restrain the patient	The patient becomes extremely agitated and bites the doctor. In the struggle he falls to the floor, fracturing a hip	The patient already thinks that he is being attacked. He attempts to protect himself, and injures the doctor and/or himself if adequate steps to prevent injury (described on pp. 266-267) are not taken
Attempt to sedate the patient with a barbiturate, benzodiazepine or anti-psychotic drug	The patient's confusion and agitation increase	Agents that depress cortical or RAS activity worsen the primary disorder of consciousness. The patient's anxiety and agitation then increase in response to further depressed brain function

A SUCCESSFUL APPROACH

When the physician communicates a calm, confident sense of control, the patient often is immediately reassured and is likely to relax:

Dr: Mr. O., no one is going to hurt you. You're safe here.

Pt: It's not safe...I'm in danger...they want to kill me.

Dr: You're in _____ hospital, on the medical floor. I'm Dr. _____ and I'll see that you aren't hurt.

Pt: There are too many of them...It's not safe.

Dr: You're safe here. You came to the hospital because you had a heart attack and we're here to protect you and take care of you. Go back to your bed now so I can examine you.

Pt: Is it all right?

Dr: It's all right. Now come on back to your bed and sit down.

Pt: I don't know...(but returns to his bed)

The physician has firmly directed the patient, adding a few statements to orient him and to correct the memory defect the doctor assumes to be present. Because the patient is frightened and confused, the doctor has had to repeat his reassurances a few times before the patient was sufficiently reassured to begin to cooperate. Since the patient may forget this helpful interaction with the physician, similar comments may have to be repeated during the course of the examination, or even for as long as the OBS is present.

DIAGNOSIS OF OBS: THE SHORT MENTAL STATUS EXAM

Any hospitalized patient who develops a change in mental functioning should be thought of as having an organic brain syndrome until proved otherwise, as should any outpatient with a personality change that is sudden or unexplained by obvious current psychosocial stresses. The possible presence of OBS is explored with the short mental status exam (MSE). The short MSE, the psychological equivalent of the physical exam, is a survey of cognitive function that can raise the suspicion or confirm the presence of an organic brain syndrome. It should be applied to all patients in whom OBS is a possibility.

The short MSE is a collection of tests, designed to examine the following functions:

1. Level of consciousness. Organic brain syndromes, especially when they are acute, are accompanied by a fluctuating level of awareness ranging from alertness, to mild confusion, obtundation, and stupor.

2. Attention. Difficulty attending to simple tasks may be present in OBS, although anxiety or depression also may interfere with the ability to attend to a variety of problems. If a patient is not paying attention or cooperating, responses to other MSE tests are difficult to interpret.

3. Orientation. Time sense is the first to be lost in OBS, followed by orientation to place. Disorientation to person without disorientation to time and place and a severe memory deficit rarely is caused by an organic disturbance.

4. Memory. Deficits in recent memory, often with intact immediate and remote memory, frequently are apparent in OBS.

5. Learning of new information. The ability to learn and retain new information, which is dependent on attention and recent memory, often is impaired in OBS. Patients who do not pay attention also do poorly on tests of new learning.

6. Serial subtractions. Subtracting 7 or 3 from 100, or counting backward, tests several functions, including attention, short-term memory, and calculating ability. Anxiety, disinterest, low intelligence or educational level, preoccupation with something else, or dyscalculia also can interfere with the ability to perform this task.

While anxiety or depression can interfere with performance on any one of the MSE tasks, difficulty with all or most of them, especially if the patient's performance fluctuates on serial examinations, strongly suggests that an OBS is present. Because of the fluctuating nature of delirium and the imprecise nature of the MSE, a normal MSE on one occasion does not rule out organic brain disease. Inconsistency from one examination to the next is more characteristic of organic than of functional disturbances.

APPLICATION OF THE SHORT MSE

The MSE may be introduced by saying: "I have a number of questions that I usually ask my patients to test their memory and concentration. Some may seem very easy and others difficult. Please try as hard as you can."

Pay attention first to the patient's level of alertness. Is he consistently alert, or does he seem to drift off from time to time and to have difficulty paying attention? Look for the characteristic fluctuation in responses to MSE tasks in the cooperative patient. Start with easy questions, making them gradually more difficult. If the patient becomes frustrated, reassure him and encourage him to proceed. However, be alert to the possibility of precipitating a "catastrophic reaction" (complete emotional breakdown)that occurs if the patient is forced to face the extent of his cognitive deficits too quickly.

The application of specific tests of the short MSE is discussed below.

1. Perception of cognitive difficulties. Even before a dificit is demonstrated, the patient may be aware of problems with his thinking or memory, becoming lost easily, or other difficulties that suggest an OBS.

2. Orientation to time and place. The physician may begin testing for orientation to time by asking the patient how long he has been in the hospital. If the patient responds with a vague answer such as, "oh, a long time," he may be evading the question. The clinician then should gently insist that the patient be more precise in stating the year, month, date and day of the week. Patients who do not know the answers to these questions may confabulate (make up) an incorrect answer. While the physician's insistence that the patient answer encourages some guessing, repeated wrong answers indicate disorientation to time.

If the patient is able to name the day, date, month
and year correctly, the doctor can ask him to tell
the time of day and to estimate the length of time
doctor and patient have been speaking. Since these
tasks are more difficult, they are more sensitive
to OBS.

Insisting that the patient attempt to answer, asking
him to be specific if he seems to evade a question,
and proceeding from general to specific questions,
also is useful in testing for orientation to place:

Dr: Do you know where you are?

Pt: Sure...in the hospital.

Dr: Which hospital?

Pt: You know, the city hospital.

Dr: Can you tell me the name of the hospital
     and the name of the ward you are on?

Orientation to place usually is lost after orientation
to time, and recovered before it, in OBS. Orientation
to person is the last function to be lost. While disorientation to person may be due to a severe memory
loss, it is not common in OBS. A patient who presents
with disorientation to person, especially if he is
oriented to time and place, is likely to be schizophrenic,
hysterical or a malingerer.

3. Attention. The patient's ability to attend to a simple
    task is tested with the letter recognition test, in
    which the doctor recites a series of randomly selected
    letters, and asks the patient to tap or otherwise
    indicate when a particular letter is mentioned. Letters
    should be spoken at the rate of about one per second,
    the target letter occurring about 25% of the time.
    For example, in the following sequence, the target
    letter is "A": O Y A Q R Z V A A B D J F U A T A E M L A.
    The patient would be asked to indicate each time the
    letter "A" is spoken. Normal individuals can complete
    a sequence of at least 40 letters without making a
    single error. Errors such as missing a letter, clapping
    when the target letter is not mentioned, or clapping
    for an incorrect letter which follows a target letter
    (perseveration) may indicate OBS.

4. Recent memory. Difficulty with recent memory should be suspected if the physician notes inconsistencies in the patient's story. It may be tested formally by telling the patient three complex items. The patient is asked to repeat these items back immediately to ensure that he is attending to the task, and then to repeat them again in about five minutes. Any items which the physician himself can remember are satisfactory, for example, a bright red carnation, 63 Broadway, and a soft, old chair. Marked difficulty remembering some or all of the items suggests OBS.

5. Learning of new information. Learning ability may be tested with the Babcock Sentence: "What this nation needs to be rich and strong is a safe, secure supply of wood." Difficulty retaining new information is suggested if the patient has to hear the sentence more than four times before he can repeat it correctly.

6. Serial subtractions. Serial subtraction of 7 or 3 from 100 tests attention, short-term memory, and calculating ability. Having ruled out dyscalculia by asking the patient to perform one or two simple calculations, the doctor may proceed as outlined below. The right-hand column explains the interaction.

Examination	*Explanation*
Dr: Now I'd like you to try to subtract some numbers for me.	
Pt: I've never been very good at math...	The patient who anticipates difficulty with the task often tries to evade it with a disclaimer.
Dr: Please try anyway. I'd like you to subtract 7 from 100 and then 7 from each answer you get, for as long as you can.	Most patients with a junior high school education should be able to perform this task.
Pt: 100, 93 (long pause), 86 ...	Patients with OBS may take an exceptionally long time to perform the task, even if they get the right answers.

Examination	*Explanation*
Dr: Go on	
Pt: Where was I - oh yes 70, 76, 79 ...	The patient forgot the task. He now confabulates (makes up) an answer ,(70), and starts to count forward instead of backward.
76, 70, 70, 76 ...	The patient now perseverates (repeats a previous answer).
69, 62, 55 ...	He again begins subtracting correctly.

If the patient cannot perform this task at all, he can be asked
to subtract 3 from 100, or to count backward from 50. The fluctuating
disturbance seen in OBS is characterized by performing well, followed
by difficulty concentrating and forgetting the previous answer or the
task itself. The patient may then perseverate and confabulate his
answers, and once again perform well. It is the fluctuating difficulty
with the task, not the correctness of the answers, that suggests OBS.

SUBTLE PRESENTATIONS OF OBS

When a patient develops an abrupt change in thinking, emotions,
or behavior in the absence of a past history of a similar disturbance
and on short MSE is found to have a fluctuating disturbance of attention,
orientation and short-term memory, as well as decreased new learning
and impaired serial subtractions, the doctor is justified in making a
diagnosis of OBS. Often, however, the disorder develops insiduously
and the short MSE may be entirely normal in a patient with a definite
OBS. This is especially likely to occur in patients with above
average intelligence who are able to compensate for disorders of alertness, attention, orientation or memory which are not yet profound. The
doctor should suspect OBS in patients in whom one or more of the following complaints are part of the presenting picture:

1. Vague complaints from the patient or his family
   that he "isn't up to par"

2. Intellectual deterioration

3. Multiple complaints

4. Difficulty concentrating or remembering

5. Subtle changes in personality, especially if accompanied by depression, apathy or emotional lability

6. Errors in judgment at home or at work

7. Uncharacteristic irrational or impulsive behavior, including suicidal and homicidal activity

8. Uncharacteristic promiscuity

9. Inability to grasp all facets of complex problems or situations

10. Suspiciousness

11. Irritability

12. Fatigue

13. Social inappropriateness

14. Frequently getting lost

15. Incontinence

16. Chronic lateness in patients who usually are punctual

17. Insomnia

18. Repeated accidents

MSE TESTS TO UNCOVER SUBTLE OBS

When the doctor suspects organic brain disease but the short mental status exam in unrevealing, he should pursue his suspicions until he has definitely ruled out OBS. Further symptoms of OBS and MSE tests for them that can be carried out at the bedside are listed below. Since fluctuation is a hallmark of OBS, serial testing may be necessary to demonstrate an abnormality.

1. Concrete thinking commonly accompanies deteriorating brain function. It is demonstrated on MSE by an inability to abstract when proverb or similarity interpretation is tested (pp 86-88). For example, when the patient is asked to give the most general meaning of "a rolling stone gathers no moss," he

might reply "because it keeps on rolling." When asked
how a table and a chair are alike, he might answer
"they both have four legs" instead of "they are both
pieces of furniture." Such answers are particularly
indicative of OBS if the patient has previously held
a position requiring complex abstract thinking and
does not exhibit idiosyncratic thinking that might
indicate schizophrenia.

2. Constructional apraxia is the inability to perform
   a constructional task when the necessary motor and
   sensory pathways are intact. It usually is due to
   diffuse brain disease or to disease localized to
   either parietal lobe, especially on the nondominant
   side. Some patients with mild diffuse brain disease
   without severe structural damage to the posterior
   right hemisphere may not have constructional apraxia.
   Constructional apraxia is tested as follows:

   -The patient is first asked to copy figures
    drawn by the doctor. Any figure may be used,
    as long as the physician is familiar with
    the way in which patients with and without
    organic brain disease copy them. It is a
    good idea to have the patient copy at least
    one three dimensional figure. Some commonly
    used figures are:

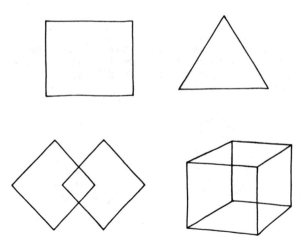

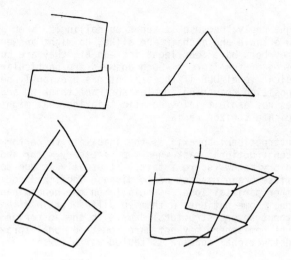

The figures (above) of the patient with OBS are distorted,
rotated and fragmented, with particular difficulty
copying angles and three dimensional aspects of the
drawings. The organic brain disease patient may draw
his figures very close to those of the examiner.

- Next, the patient draws a few figures <u>on command</u>
  (without copying). Again, any figure will do, for
  example a clock with numbers on the face and the hands
  pointing to 5:00. The patient with OBS may draw a
  clock that looks like this:

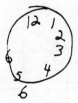

3. <u>Impaired ability to perform simple motor tasks</u> occurs
    in diffuse cortical and frontal lobe disease.
    Patients with organic brain disease should
    have little trouble with the following tasks
    after one or two tries:

    -<u>Hand clapping</u>. The examiner asks the patient
    to start clapping his hands with the doctor,
    and to stop the instant he stops. Difficulty
    starting or stopping may be present in organic
    brain disease.

    -<u>Palm-edge-fist test</u>. The patient claps his
    palm, edge of hand, and fist against the opposite
    palm. After he has practiced a few times, he
    is asked to continue for 15 seconds. Difficulty
    starting or stopping, or motor perseveration
    (e.g., repeating the edge, instead of moving
    on to the fist) suggest organic brain disease.

4. <u>Aphasias</u> (or dysphasias) usually are caused by disease
    of the hemisphere dominant for speech. To uncover
    aphasia, the examiner first listens to the aphasic
    patient speak. Then the patient is asked to read a
    few sentences, say from a newspaper or book, and
    the doctor decides whether his speech is fluent
    or nonfluent.

    -<u>Nonfluent Aphasia</u> is sparse and agrammatical,
    contains many pauses, and consists mostly of
    nouns. For example, in describing what brought
    him to the hospital, a patient might say, "I...
    hospital...day..."

    -<u>Fluent Aphasia</u> flows easily but because it
    contains many paraphasias (abnormal words
    that substitute for the correct word and resemble
    it in some way), it is difficult to understand.
    For example, when asked to describe his symptom,
    a patient might say, "Well, they start where...
    it's a harp main...

The physician can screen for aphasia by asking the
patient to:

    -<u>Understand</u> a few simple statements (e.g., "go
    to the table and get a glass of water").

-Repeat a few simple phrases (e.g., "no, if's, and's or but's").

-Name a few objects, preferably with more than one part to the name, (e.g., neck tie, belt buckle, and fountain pen).

Any combination of difficulty understanding, repeating, or naming that cannot easily be explained on the basis of intelligence, education, or cultural background suggests that aphasia, and therefore organic brain disease, is present.

5. Parietal lobe dysfunction may cause symptoms that mimic psychiatric disease. A screening exam tests for:

-Dressing Apraxia. The patient is asked to put on his shirt or bathrobe after it has been turned inside-out. Difficulty performing this task when motor and sensory pathways are intact is strongly suggestive of OBS.

-Topographical Memory. The patient is asked to describe a few simple directions (e.g., from his house to the grocery store) and directions from his home city to various other locations, e.g., to Canada, Mexico, and Europe, and to label a map. Difficulty with these tasks that cannot be explained by education, intelligence, or obvious psychotic or idiosyncratic thinking, indicates brain disease. (Some demented patients who repeatedly get lost have a disturbance of topographical memory).

CONFIRMATION OF THE DIAGNOSIS

If the presence of OBS is suspected but not well documented, or if the doctor wishes to confirm the diagnosis and begin to investigate etiology, the following special procedures can be considered:

1. EEG. The electroencephalogram may become slower than the usual alpha rhythm (8-13 cps). At times, the predominant rhythm may become faster, especially if centrally acting drugs have been taken. While an abnormal EEG indicates brain dysfunction,

many patients with OBS have a normal tracing.
Serial recordings may demonstrate slowing of
the predominant rhythm with a
worsening of the patient's state.

2. <u>C-T Scan</u>. Computerized tomography is of value in
   demonstrating a number of brain lesions, including
   cerebral atrophy, hydrocephalus, and intracerebral
   hematomas.

3. <u>Neuropsychological testing</u>. The Halstead-Reitan
   Battery is a day-long series of complex motor,
   perceptual and cognitive tests. It can be useful
   in confirming the presence of OBS, localizing the
   lesion, and determining whether the disorder is
   static or progressive. This test also can be useful
   in documenting types and degrees of deficits that
   are likely to affect the patient's everyday
   functioning.

AN INTEGRATED APPROACH TO THE DIAGNOSIS
OF ORGANIC BRAIN SYNDROMES

OBS should be ruled out in any patient who develops a change
in thinking, mood, or behavior. While depression and anxiety are
the most common presenting complaints, symptoms vary from apathy
to neurotic symptoms to euhporia to psychosis. Onset may be sudden
or insidious, and the patient's reaction to the primary cognitive
impairment depends in large part on his pre-existing personality.

When OBS is a possibility, the workup may be efficiently
approached in this way:

1. The short mental status exam is a good screening
   tool. If orientation, short-term memory and
   serial subtractions are impaired, OBS is likely
   and a diagnostic workup aimed at determining its
   etiology should begin.

2. If OBS is suspected and the short MSE is equivocal,
   further bedside testing for concrete thinking,
   constructional apraxia, aphasia, parietal lobe
   dysfunction and inability to perform simple motor
   tasks may be performed.

3. Because symptoms tend to fluctuate, repeated
    testing may be necessary to uncover OBS.

4. Neurological exam may uncover "hard" or "soft"
    lateralizing signs, strengthening the impression
    of organic brain disease and suggesting
    directions for further workup.

5. The diagnosis can be confirmed, and etiology and
    degree of impairment investigated, with EEG,
    C-T scan, and neuropsychological testing.

ETIOLOGY

While _any_ disorder that directly or indirectly affects the
brain can produce an organic brain syndrome, some conditions are
especially likely to be causes of OBS in a general hospital
population. These include:

1. Drug intoxication. Many prescription and non-
    prescription drugs affect cerebral function,
    and intoxication is an especially likely cause
    of OBS in older patients with pre-existing marginal
    brain reserves who are receiving multiple medications
    and in patients who are being treated by more than
    one physician. Some medications directly disturb
    cortical metabolism (e.g., anticholinergics), some
    depress cortical or reticular activating system
    activity (e.g., psychotropic drugs), and some can
    produce OBS as an idiosyncratic reaction (e.g.,
    aspirin). Drug interactions also may produce OBS
    (e.g., addictive effect of two anticholinergic drugs
    such as chlorpromazine and amitriptyline). Even
    reliable patients may not admit to all the medications
    (including over-the-counter preparations) they are
    taking and a drug history may have to be obtained
    from family members and other physicians or from a
    blood screen.

2. Alcohol or drug withdrawal. Withdrawal from alcohol,
    barbiturates, minor tranquilizers or sedative-hypnotics
    can produce an acute OBS within hours to days after
    the patient is hospitalized and stops taking the
    drug. Because many patients do not volunteer an
    accurate drug and alcohol history, a history of the
    use of the substances also should be obtained from

relatives and friends, and inquiries about substance use made repeatedly. This diagnosis can be even more difficult when the patient secretly continues to drink or take a drug while in the hospital and only starts to withdraw when his supply runs out, or when he is taking a long acting drug (e.g., a benzodiazepine) that produces a delayed abstinence syndrome. Withdrawal should be considered in any patient who develops an acute OBS within a few hours to a week after admission to the hospital   (see pp. 138-140).

3. Organ failure. Cardiorespiratory disorders that result in altered cerebral blood flow and/or oxygenation (e.g., congestive heart failure, pulmonary embolism) are common causes of OBS in patients on the coronary care unit. Failure of any other organ system (especially liver and kidney) also may produce an OBS.

4. Infection. Central nervous system infections, or the effects on the brain of systemic or localized infections, should be suspected as causes of OBS in patients at risk of developing such infections (e.g., wound infection in postoperative patients or brain abcesses in immunosuppressed patients). Syphilis, while uncommon, may present as an acute or chronic OBS.

5. Metabolic and endocrine disturbances. These disturbances should be searched for when other obvious causes of OBS are not found. For example, thyroid dysfunction or hypoglycemia can produce acute or chronic brain syndromes in the absence of other physical findings. Hypocalcemia produces anxiety, agitation or mania while hypercalcemia causes depression, with or without obvious MSE changes. Appropriate laboratory studies are essential to making the diagnosis, and blood sugar, serum calciums and thyroid function tests are indicated in organic brain disease of unknown etiology.

6. Ion and acid-base disturbances. Water intoxication and disturbances in mineral or electrolyte disturbance occasionally present as OBS.

7. CNS disease. Any CNS disease can produce OBS due
    to alteration of brain function. Seizure disorders,
    traumatic and post-traumatic states (e.g., subdural
    hematoma), degenerative diseases, normal pressure
    hydrocephalus, and tumors are among the more common
    neurological causes of OBS.

8. Systemic diseases. Most systemic disease can affect
    the brain to produce acute or chronic OBS. Lupus
    cerebritis is a well-known example.

Unless otherwise indicated by the history or physical findings,
the initial workup should investigate these likely possibilities
first. If the workup is unrevealing, less likely causes should be
investigated (e.g., occult neoplasm, heavy metal poisoning, etc.).

HOSPITAL MANAGEMENT OF THE DELIRIOUS PATIENT

The primary goal in the approach to organic brain syndrome is
to diagnose and treat the underlying disease state. While the workup
is proceeding, the patient's emotional and behavioral reaction to his
cognitive impairment usually can be managed using the techniques
listed in the left-hand column below. These techniques, which are
further analyzed on the right, temporarily compensate for the underlying disturbance of consciousness. For example, if the patient
does not remember where he is, this information is repeatedly
supplied to him. The more he knows, the less frightened the patient
is of a situatuion that he does not understand and his agitation
decreases. The patient's nurses, who have frequent, regular contact
with him, are often in the best position to carry out the measures
described below and to repeat them frequently in order to compensate
for the patient's poor memory.

Treatment Plan	_Analysis_
Explain to the patient that he is confused because of the effects of a medical illness on his brain, and that the doctor will do his best to diagnose and treat the problem	Many patients do not appreciate the obvious reason for their distress until it is explained to them. They are reassured when they are provided with an understandable explanation

Treatment Plan	*Analysis*
Remind the patient where he is	When disorientation to place is decreased, the patient is less frightened
Remind the patient of the names of doctors and nurses, and of the fact that they are taking care of him for a specific illness	If the patient has forgotten that the people around him are hospital personnel, he may assume because he is in pain and frightened, that these "strangers" are trying to hurt him
Place a clock, calendar and radio in the patient's room. Keep the lights on in the patient's room	A constant source of information that orients the patient, reduces anxiety and agitation due to the patient's not knowing the date or where he is
Put the patient in a room that is close to the nursing station	This location makes frequent visits by nursing staff easier, providing them with an opportunity to orient and reassure the patient
Avoid frequent changes of doctors and nurses	Because of his memory disturbance, the patient has difficulty keeping track of a large number of care-takers. He is confused and frightened by people he does not remember
Restrict visitors to close friends and relatives	Seeing people the patient does not remember is confusing and frightening to him
Encourage unrestricted visits by relatives and close friends	The patient is reassured by familiar people. Familiar visitors also can help to reassure and orient the patient when nursing staff is unavailable

APPROACH TO MEDICATION

When structure, reassurance and orientation are not sufficient or when there is not enough time for them to take effect, medications must be used to calm agitated patients with organic brain syndromes. Unfortunately, many commonly used tranquilizing drugs further depress cortical and reticular activating system activity, increasing the primary disorder of consciousness. This makes the patient more anxious, and increases agitation, which is a behavioral response to anxiety. For example, while low doses of anti-anxiety drugs (e.g., diazepam) may produce initial improvement, their long half-life results in a build-up of blood levels, with eventual worsening of symptoms if they are prescribed for too long a period of time. If the dose then is increased further, the patient's symptoms may become still worse until he is "snowed". The same is true of sedating anti-psychotic drugs (e.g., chlorpromazine). Barbiturates (e.g., amytal) can produce marked CNS depression and are especially dangerous if intracranial disease is present.

In patients with acute OBS, agitation usually is episodic, occurring when the patient's primary disorder of consciousness is worse (e.g., at night). The behavioral disturbance is worsened by anything that further impairs consciousness or requires more cognitive abilities than are possessed by the patient (e.g., fever, new surroundings, or a change of doctors). These factors often make regularly scheduled doses of medication inefficient in controlling agitation.

An approach that takes both the fluctuating nature of the underlying disturbance and the tendency of many tranquilizing drugs to impair consciousness further into account suggests the following guidelines:

1. Many cases of OBS in the general hospital are due to the effects of multiple drugs on the patient's sensorium. A good first step therefore is to stop all drugs not essential to the patient's treatment.

2. Good results have been achieved with nonsedating antipsychotic drugs (e.g., haloperidol). These should be prescribed:

    -episodically to correspond with episodes of agitation (e.g., if the patient is always worse at 3 AM, give the medication at 2 AM)

-regularly if periods of agitation cannot
be predicted

-in <u>low</u> doses (e.g., 0.5-2 mg haloperidol
up <u>to</u> QID)

3. Antihistamines (e.g., hydroxyzine or diphenhydramine)
also may be useful as tranquilizers or sleeping pills.
In a dose of 100 mg, they also may be utilized to
sedate an anxious patient for an EEG, as they do not
affect·the predominant rhythm.

4. Acute OBS due to withdrawal from alcohol, sedatives
or tranquilizers is treated with high doses of
antianxiety drugs or barbiturates over a short
period of time. A test dose of phenobarbital or
pentobarbital differentiates abstinence syndromes
from other causes of OBS (see pp. 145-146).

5. Drugs that decrease agitation in patients with anxiety
due to "functional" disorders but worsen it in OBS
sometimes may be used to differentiate organic brain
disease from non-organic conditions. When differential
diagnosis is very difficult, and the physician is
<u>certain</u> that the patient does not have a space-
occupying brain lesion, a test dose of amytal sodium
(100-200 mg) may be given parenterally. Because the
barbiturate further depresses brain function, patients
with OBS usually worsen, while many patients with
anxiety due to non-organic causes improve.

6. Physical restraints may be used until the patient can
be medicated, to allow medication time to work, or if
medication is unsuccessful.

7. Since high doses of antidepressants can depress CNS
activity, they may worsen the primary disorder of
consciousness and actually worsen the depression in
patients with organic brain syndromes. Patients who
are acutely depressed due to OBS can be expected to
improve when the underlying disorder is treated
and should not be given antidepressants.

The following additional guidelines apply to the medication
of dementia:

1. Agitation in demented patients often is related
to worsening of the underlying disease process,
development of an intercurrent illness (e.g., a

mild infection) that leads to a breakdown of
marginally compensated brain function, or a change
in environment or caretakers (e.g., a new nurse)
that the patient is unable to handle. These
possibilities should be investigated before the
patient is medicated.

2. The measures described for managing acute agitation
in delirious patients also apply in dementia.

3. Because they depress brain function, standard
sleeping pills are likely to produce paradoxical
excitement in demented patients and elderly people
with diminished brain reserves. If leaving a light
on at night does not help the patient to get to sleep,
an antihistamine (e.g., diphenhydramine 25-50 mg),
L-tryptophan, or a low dose of haloperidol
(e.g., 0.5 mg) may prove helpful.

4. When chronic depression complicates a chronic
organic brain syndrome and does not respond to
support and psychotherapy, low doses of tricyclic
antidepressants (e.g., 10-30 mg/day of imipramine)
may be prescribed.

5. A number of medications, particularly neurotransmitter
precursors, have been used in attempts to improve
cognitive function in Alzheimer's disease and other
dementias of the elderly. Of these, choline and
L-dopa have been shown to improve cognition somewhat,
although this improvement is not clinically significant.
Lecithin, a choline precursor, may prove useful in
long-term treatment. Hydergine, a combination of
ergot drugs, may produce modest improvement in
depression and self-care in some demented patients.
It must be administered for 3-6 months (at a dose
of 1 mg TID) before it can be said not to be
working.

6. Assaultive outbursts in brain-injured patients
have been treated successfully with propranolol,
60-320 mg/day, when other treatments have failed.

7. Even though emotional disturbances in many patients
with organic brain syndromes can be managed without
medication, the physician should not feel uncomfortable
about prescribing drugs when they are necessary.

PSYCHIATRIC SIDE EFFECTS OF DRUGS USED
IN MEDICAL PRACTICE

In addition to acute organic brain syndromes, a number of medications may produce mental symptoms that can be mistaken for psychiatric problems. Important side effects of commonly prescribed medications are summarized in the left-hand column below, and some drugs that produce them are listed in the middle column. Comments can be found in the right-hand column.

Symptom	Medications	Comments
Depression	corticosteroids; ACTH minor tranquilizers barbiturates clonazepam narcotics amphetamines disulfiram anticonvulsants indomethacin isoniazid L-dopa methyldopa; reserpine halothane niridazole propranolol nalidixic acid phenylephrine vinblastine asparaginase	Risk of suicide may be significant
Hallucinations	amantadine anticonvulsants antihistamines anticholinergics baclofen bromocriptine chloroquine cimeditine corticosteroids; ACTH cycloserine digitalis disopyramide indomethacin isoniazid metrizamide	Symptoms may be accompanied by other symptoms of delirium and may not be dose related

Symptom	Medications	Comments
Hallucinations (continued)	nalidixic acid propranolol quinacrine thiabendazole penicillin G	
	minor tranquilizers barbiturates amphetamines ephedrine phenylephrine methylphenidate	Usually due to intoxication or withdrawal when excessive doses are given
	L-dopa	Risk increases with prolonged use
	procainamide vincristine	Hallucinations are rare
	ketamine	See below
Mania	baclofen	Symptoms usually appear after sudden withdrawal
	bromocriptine	Symptoms may continue after the drug is withdrawn
	corticosteroids; ACTH	Symptoms may appear at high or low doses
	niridazole	Symptoms appear at higher doses
	L-dopa phenelzine digitalis	Other affective symptoms also may appear, usually with higher doses
Nightmares	amantadine baclofen	After withdrawal
	digitalis	Usually with high plasma levels

Symptom	Medications	Comments
Nightmares (continued)	ketamine	Also produces hallucinations, crying, changes in body image and acute OBS
	L-dopa pentazocine propranolol	Usually after a dosage increase
Paranoia	asparaginase bromocriptine corticosteroids, ACTH cycloserine	See above Anxiety, depression, and delirium also are common
	amphetamines	May occur even at low doses
	digitalis indomethacin	Especially in elderly
	isonazid L-dopa	See above
	phenylephrine, ephedrine	Symptoms appears with excessive dosage
	propranolol	Symptoms appear with high or low doses
	sulindac	
Aggressive behavior	bromocriptine chloroquine dapsone diazepam disopyramide	Symptoms may appear even with low doses shortly after treatment is initiated
	digitalis	See above
	ethchlorvynol	Symptoms appear with prolonged dosage
	L-dopa	See above

Symptom	Medications	Comments
Aggressive Behavior (continued)	phenelzine	Symptoms resolve rapidly when drug is discontinued
	sulindac	See above
Anticholinergic psychosis	atropine antidepressants eye drops nose drops over-the-counter sleeping pills antihistamines scopolamine anticholinergics (e.g., benztropine, trihexyphenidyl) cyclopentolate	Delirium occurs with mydriasis, warm, dry skin, fever and tachycardia. Physostigmine 1 mg IV can be utilized diagnostically and to treat coma and severe hyperpyrexia

OUTPATIENT MANAGEMENT OF THE DEMENTED PATIENT

Delirious patients improve when the underlying disorder is treated, and usually are symptom-free when they are discharged from the hospital. In chronic organic brain disease (dementia), the underlying cause usually cannot be reversed and the patient must continue to live with some degree of cognitive impairment. In addition to measures that reduce emotional and behavioral reactions to the primary disorder, the patient and his family must be helped to adjust to his disability. The following guidelines are useful in the outpatient management of chronic OBS:

1. Convey appropriate optimism that while the patient's disease cannot be cured, much can be done to help him to adapt to his reduced mental capacity and to make the most of life.

2. Assess the patient's capabilities and weaknesses in order to help him to make realistic plans for himself. For example, an electronics engineer with mild chronic OBS may experience confusion, anxiety, and depression if he attempts to continue work which is beyond his conceptual abilities.

However, he may be able to perform more limited
tasks successfully.

3. Discuss the patient's loss of cognitive abilities
   openly with the patient and his family, facilitating
   grieving for lost mental functions in the patient
   and loss of the person they once knew in the family
   (see pp. 176-185).

4. Sudden changes in mental functioning may signify the
   development of an acute OBS complicating the chronic
   disorder. The new problem may be treatable and
   its etiology should be actively investigated.

5. Maintain as consistent an environment as possible,
   minimizing changes in caretakers, furnishings, etc.

6. Enlist the aid of the family in managing emotional
   and behavioral reactions to OBS. Measures such
   as keeping the lights on in the patient's room,
   providing him with a calendar, and correcting
   disordered memory and orientation are useful at
   home as well as in the hospital.

7. Follow guidelines to the use of medication outlined
   on pp. 102-104. Avoid prescribing any drugs (including
   aspirin) that are not essential to the patient's
   health. Ask the patient if he is taking tonics,
   over-the-counter preparations, and other substances
   that he may not consider medications but that may
   be worsening chronic OBS.

8. Ensure that all discussions and directions are in
   simple, concrete language and are repeated frequently.

9. Do not assume that older patients who develop a change
   in thinking, feeling or behavior are demented. Many
   are suffering from depression resulting from isolation
   from loved ones, unresolved grief over lost functions
   and loved ones (especially in older patients) and
   hopelessness in caretakers.

10. Ensure adequate hydration, nutrition, and intake of
    vitamins. The patient may not remember to eat or
    drink well, and even minimal malnutrition can aggravate
    the effects of the underlying disease on the
    patient's brain.

11. Discuss with the patient and his family the necessity of avoiding alcohol and sedating and tranquilizing drugs, which may further impair brain function.

12. While supporting efforts to maintain the patient outside of a nursing home, help the family to recognize when their resources are exhausted and placement away from the home is necessary. Deal with feelings of failure and guilt, as well as relief, that arise in conjunction with this issue.

DIFFERENTIAL DIAGNOSIS

Organic brain disease can be confused with any psychiatric disorder. In most cases, but not inevitably, responses to MSE and other tests are abnormal in OBS and normal in functional disturbances. Disorders that are commonly confused with OBS are listed below, opposite salient differentiating features.

Psychiatric Diagnosis	*Salient Differentiating Features*
Schizophrenia's hallucinations, delusions, and unusual behavior may seem similar to disturbances in perception and thinking seen in delirium	-Hallucinations and delusions are more bizarre and removed from real-life experiences, and more complex, in schizophrenia -Schizophrenic hallucinations are more likely to be auditory and less likely to be accompanied by illusions -The schizophrenic patient is more likely to have a past history and family history of schizophrenia -The onset of symptoms is more sudden and unexpected in OBS -Hallucinations and delusions in delirium fluctuate, while schizophrenic symptoms tend to be more consistent

Psychiatric Diagnosis	*Salient Differentiating Features*
Depression is common in response to the primary disorder of consciousness in OBS; severely depressed patients may complain of difficulty with concentration and memory that mimic dementia ("depressive pseudo-dementia")	-Vegetative signs usually are absent in OBS -Depressed patients with memory disturbances have a mood disturbance that is greater than the degree of memory loss -Special tests (e.g., EEG) are normal in depression but may be abnormal in OBS -Guilt and lowered self-esteem are more prominent in depression -Depressed patients may respond favorably to standard doses of anti-depressants, while symptoms of patients with OBS are likely to worsen
Hypochondriasis may seem to be present in patients with chronic OBS who have multiple somatic complaints; hypochondriacal patients may develop organic brain syndromes if they are overmedicated	-Symptoms are more likely to fluctuate in OBS -MSE is normal in hypochondriasis -Illness claiming behavior is not a prominent symptom of OBS
Hysteria may produce memory loss that is difficult to differentiate from OBS	-Memory loss in hysteria is specific to areas of emotional conflict -Disorientation to person may accompany a mild memory disturbance in hysteria -Memory loss occurs in response to an emotional stress -The hysterical patient is less likely to be worried by symptoms ("la belle indifference") -Fluctuation is less obvious in hysteria
Anxiety states can interfere with the patient's ability to attend to MSE tasks; many OBS patients suffer significant anxiety	-If the anxious patient is helped to calm down and pay attention, his performance on MSE tests improves -Anti-anxiety drugs and barbiturates temporarily improve neurotic anxiety, while they worsen anxiety due to OBS -Special tests (EEG, etc.) are normal in patients with neurotic anxiety

Psychiatric Diagnosis	*Salient Differentiating Features*
Malingering occasionally is confused with OBS when the patient simulates confusion or memory loss for obvious gain	-Abnormalities are less likely to fluctuate in malingering -MSE findings reflect the patient's concept of OBS (e.g., disorientation to person without disorientation to time and place) -Confusion is less prominent when the patient thinks that he is not being watched
Mania may be very difficult to distinguish from affective disturbances caused by a chronic organic brain syndrome without obvious cognitive disturbance or intellectural deterioration (organic affective syndrome)	-Careful MSE and special testing are abnormal -An organic disorder is suspected from the history, physical examination or laboratory studies -Symptoms worsen with antipsychotic drugs or lithium
Personality disorders, especially those involving loss of impulse control, may be simulated by chronic organic brain disorders (organic personality syndrome).	-Emotional lability or apathy are apparent -A history of an organic disorder that can affect brain function is present -Subtle signs of dementia are present -Special MSE and laboratory tests are abnormal

USE OF THE PSYCHIATRIST

As a cognitive, emotional, and behavioral reaction to an underlying medical or surgical disorder, OBS usually is managed on the medical or surgical floor or in the primary physician's office. The psychiatrist can be invaluable in making a diagnosis and developing a plan to manage the patient's behavior.

The physician should consult with the psychiatrist if:

1. The diagnosis is not clear

2. The physician wishes further understanding of the ways in which the patient's personality influences his reaction to the primary disorder of consciousness

3. The doctor's approach to managing the patient is unsuccessful

4. The patient may be suicidal or homicidal

5. The physician wishes assistance in choosing a medication

The physician should <u>refer the patient to the psychiatrist if</u>:

1. The patient's behavior makes management on an open medical floor difficult or impossible (e.g., he needs constant attention to prevent suicide)

2. The doctor is unable or unwilling to manage emotional reactions to chronic OBS

3. The family's reaction to the patient's condition, especially if it is irreversible, is complicated or extreme

4. An organic brain syndrome complicates or is complicated by another psychiatric disorder (e.g., severe or chronic depression)

REFERENCES

Benson DF, Blumer O: Psychiatric Aspects of Neurologic Disease.
New York, Grune and Stratton, 1975.

Benson DF, Geschwind N: Psychiatric Conditions Associated with Focal
Lesions of the CNS, In: Arieti S, Reiser MF (eds): American Handbook of Psychiatry (2nd Ed) Vol. 4. New York, Basic Books, 1975.
pp 208-243.

Engel G, Romano J: Delirium, A Syndrome of Cerebral Insufficiency.
J. Chronic Dis 1959; 9:260.

Heller S, Kornfeld DS: Delirium and Related Problems. In: Reiser
MF (ed): American Handbook of Psychiatry (2nd Ed) Vol. 4.
New York, Basic Books, 1975. pp 43-66.

Jacobs JW, Bernhard MR, Delgado A, et al: Screening for Organic Mental
Syndromes in The Medically Ill. Ann Intern Med 1977; 86:40.

Lipowski ZL: Delirium. Springfield, Ill., C.C.Thomas, 1980.

Medical Letter: Drugs that Cause Psychiatric Symptoms. Medical Letter
1981; 23:9.

McEvoy JP: Organic Brain Syndromes. Ann Intern Med 1981; 95:212.

Strub RL, Black FW: The Mental Status Examination in Neurology.
Philadelphia, FA Davis, 1977.

Wells CE: Dementia Philadelphia, FA Davis, 1971.

Chapter Five

SUBSTANCE ABUSE

by Stephen L. Dilts, M.D., Ph.D.

Substance abuse refers to the use of psychoactive drugs, including alcohol, to the extent of <u>significant interference with the user's physical, social, and/or emotional well-being</u>. It is characterized by preoccupation with the drug and loss of control over its use. If the quantity and duration of abuse is sufficient, physical dependence may develop, with tolerance and risk of a withdrawal syndrome when drug use is terminated. As physical dependence progresses, higher doses are required to achieve the same effect and prevent withdrawal symptoms, and the abuser becomes more and more preoccupied with obtaining an increasing supply of the drug. Psychological dependence may develop concomitantly, with repeated failures at attempts to stop drug use, an uncontrollable urge to use the drug, and a life centered around the drug. Concepts important to an understanding of substance abuse include:

Drug Abuse: A pathological pattern of use of a drug (e.g., inability to decrease intake, intoxication during the day, etc.), causing impairment of social or occupational functioning (e.g., loss of job, divorce, arrests, etc.) and lasting at least one month

Drug Dependence: A severe form of drug abuse that is accompanied by physical dependence, evidenced by tolerance and/or withdrawal

Tolerance: The requirement for a higher dose of a drug than was originally required to achieve a given effect, or the phenomenon of diminished effect with the same dose

Withdrawal: Appearance of specific physical symptoms (abstinence syndrome) when drug intake is decreased or stopped suddenly

Alcoholism: Abuse of and dependence on alcohol

Addiction: Extreme drug abuse in which the activities
of obtaining and using a drug totally pervade the life
of the user

Anti-anxiety Agents: Drugs that reduce anxiety, e.g.,
benzodiazepines

Sedative-hypnotic Drugs: Central nervous system
depressants that are used to produce sleep, e.g.,
secobarbital, gluethimide

Although the primary clinician often encounters patients who abuse
anti-anxiety drugs, sleeping pills, or analgesics, even more substance
abuse in clinical practice involves alcohol. Common patterns of abuse
include widely scattered binges, weekend binges, and continuous drinking. Unsuccessful attempts to stop drinking, blackouts, and drinking
despite physical complications also are common, and loss of job, legal
problems, violence while intoxicated and disruption of social relationships are equally frequent. Alcoholics frequently begin to develop
problems related to alcohol abuse within the first five years of regular
drinking. Psychological complications include anxiety and depression,
with a high rate of suicide. Physical complications are found in all
body systems.

Alcohol abuse is estimated to affect 10% of the adult population.
Men are affected four to five times as frequently as women, although
it is thought that many women are not diagnosed as alcoholics because
their drinking is easier to hide. The following factors place a
person at high risk for alcohol abuse:

1. Family history of alcoholism

2. Family history of teetotalism

3. History of alcoholism in the spouse or
    the spouse's family

Undiagnosed alcohol abusers may present with vague gastrointestinal
symptoms, poorly explained injuries, organic brain syndromes, or
unexpected withdrawal symptoms (e.g., seizures or delirium) when
hospitalized for other reasons. If the patient presents with these
problems or if interference with physical, social, or emotional well-
being is reported by the patient or his family, alcoholism can be
diagnosed even when the patient denies excessive drinking.

The next most common substance abuse problem encountered in clinical practice involves anti-anxiety drugs and sleeping pills. Daily doses two or three times higher than those usually prescribed may result in physical dependence in as little as one month. The use of 600 mg. or more per day of secobarbital or 60 mg. of diazepam or their equivalent is sufficient cause to diagnose drug abuse. Abusers of these medications frequently are doctor-shopping middle-aged housewives with vague emotional and physical complaints, but anyone may develop this problem. As in alcoholism, intoxication may result in poorly explained injuries, unexplained organic brain syndromes, and unexpected withdrawal symptoms when hospitalized. Narcotic abuse may be seen in chronically ill patients, especially those with personality disorders. Narcotic addiction is only very rarely created by administering high doses of analgesics to hospitalized acutely ill patients.

The problems encountered in handling various types of substance abusers are similar, as is their management. Since alcoholism is most common, it will be the focus of the initial discussion in this chapter to illustrate principles of treatment.

CLUES TO THE DIAGNOSIS OF ALCOHOLISM

The presence of any or all of the following raises the suspicion of alcoholism:

1. High blood alcohol level (BAL) on elective admission to the hospital, especially with a normal mental status exam (indicates tolerance to alcohol)

2. Anxiety, tremulousness, tachycardia, nausea or seizures shortly after admission to the hospital (may indicate incipient withdrawal)

3. Criticism of the patient's drinking by family and friends

4. History of blackouts

5. Presence or history of unexplained injuries

6. Family history of alcoholism

7. Presence of alcoholism in the spouse

8. Family history of teetotalism

9. Arrest for driving under the influence
   of alcohol

10. Loss of several jobs in a row

11. Marital problems

12. Impotence

ENCOUNTER WITH A TYPICAL PATIENT

Mr. A. is a 44-year-old man admitted to the Medical Service for workup of epigastric pain and weight loss during the past six months. He complains of frequent headaches, tension and mild depression, which he attributes to pressures at work. He says that his appetite is poor, that he has not been sleeping well, and that things at home are not ideal. He has had similar symptoms several times over the past five years, having obtained some relief with antacids and anti-anxiety drugs, and admits to only "an occasional social drink." His mother died of cirrhosis a number of years ago.

Physical exam reveals ecchymoses on his legs. Because of an odor of alcohol on his breath, a blood alcohol level (BAL) is obtained and is reported to be 105 mg. %. Mental status exam (MSE) is normal.

During his first two days in the hospital, Mr. A seems increasingly anxious and develops tachycardia, sweating, tremulousness, and nausea. He demands that he be given tranquilizers and that "you get this show on the road so that I can get out of here, because this place is driving me crazy." Mental status exam now shows slight deficits in attention and memory. On closer questioning, Mrs. A volunteers that she thinks that her husband drinks too much. The patient denies this, saying that his wife constantly bothers him and that he never has more than a couple of beers or cocktails daily. However, at this point he admits to having had a "blackout" or two, and volunteers the information that he recently changed jobs.

Mr. A's anxiety, tachycardia, sweating, tremulousness, and nausea early in the hospitalization suggest withdrawal from alcohol, anti-

anxiety drugs or sedatives. The suggestion of a family history of
alcoholism, apparent tolerance to alcohol at admission (high BAL without signs of intoxication on MSE) and withdrawal symptoms all point
to the diagnosis of alcoholism. His possible marital difficulties,
occupational problems, and symptoms of anxiety and depression probably
are directly related to his alcohol consumption, as are his ulcer-like
symptoms. "Blackouts," which consist of amnesia for events that
occurred when the patient was drinking, are especially suggestive of
alcoholism. Thus, alcohol is likely to be interfering with the patient's
physical, social and emotional health.

When alcohol abuse is suspected, it is important to obtain a
history of other drugs used. Since Mr. A has mentioned use of anti-
anxiety agents, more information about these medications will help to
determine whether he has a mixed pattern of abuse. However, the
patient's history is likely not entirely reliable and additional
information may have to be obtained from family members and possibly
from a toxic screen.

The first step in the treatment of any substance abuse problem is
to detoxify the patient. Even if the patient is seen in the office,
withdrawal should only take place in the hospital. Tables located at
the end of this chapter list common drugs of abuse with symptoms of
intoxication, withdrawal syndromes, and detoxification procedures
(see pp. 137-147).

After completing detoxification, Mr. A begins to ask about the
results of his tests. He is feeling better, and the physician
approaches him to tell him the diagnosis.

Pt: What did my tests show?

Dr: Well, your upper GI series was normal, but your
      blood tests showed some liver abnormalities
      caused by your drinking. Alcohol probably
      caused your stomach pain also.

Pt: I don't drink that much. I just need a little
      Librium to handle the pressure at work.

Dr: But Mr. A, you're an alcoholic. You'll just
      become addicted to the tranquilizers, too.

Pt: Alcoholic! Who do you think you're talking
      to, young man! My wife must have put you up to
      this. If she'd just get off my back, I wouldn't
      need to be here in the first place.

Dr: Well, Mr. A, I'm the doctor here and I'm
     telling you that you're an alcoholic. If
     you don't realize that, you'll just get
     sicker.

THE PHYSICIAN'S REACTION TO HIS PATIENT

Alcoholics frequently elicit strong reactions in their doctors,
some of which are illustrated below. The comments in the right-hand
column elucidate the kinds of information that can be obtained from
such reactions.

Physician's Reaction	Comment
Lack of awareness of any reaction	It would be unusual to have no reaction to a patient who belittles and does not listen to the physician. This reaction may indicate that the physician feels uncomfortable being angry with the patient
Pity for the patient	Anger may be handled by changing it into another emotion in which the physician looks down on the patient with disguised contempt
Discouragement	The physician may have identified with the despair that underlies the patient's bravado, or exposure to "skid row" alcoholics in medical school may have led the physician to conclude that alcoholism is untreatable
Anger with patient	The alcoholic's hostility, egocentricity and tendency to externalize his problems make the doctor's efforts seem futile and frustrating, arousing understandable irritation

Anger at the alcoholic patient may be expressed by doctors in the form of:

1. Making hostile jokes about him

2. Overprescribing anti-anxiety drugs to keep him quiet

3. Refusing to be "manipulated" and underprescribing medications

4. Discharging the inpatient prematurely

5. Telling the patient that he will have to find another doctor

6. Ignoring the patient

7. Telling the patient that he will die immediately if he does not stop drinking

COMMON UNSUCCESSFUL APPROACHES

Following are some interventions that are commonly attempted with the alcoholic and his reactions to them. An explanation of the patient's response can be found in the right-hand column.

Physician's Approach	*Patient's Response*	*Explanation*
Attempt to convince the patient that with sufficient willpower he should be able to go home and stop drinking	The patient agrees but begins drinking 2 days after discharge	The substance abuser often ignores (denies) the magnitude of his problem and his need for help in order to protect himself from feeling worthless. He feels good about himself as long as he can convince himself that he has everything under control and the recognition

Physician's Approach	*Patient's Response*	*Explanation*
		that he is not in control makes him feel worthless. Supporting denial of the patient's inability to stop drinking makes him feel good temporarily; however, when his will-power fails he feels worse about himself and drinks even more in order to suppress increasing feelings of failure
Make the patient feel guilty about what he is doing to him-self and his family	The patient agrees that he had better quit drinking but continues to drink	Because alcoholics tend to be perfectionistic and set high standards for themselves, they already feel guilty and ashamed of their drinking. When the patient's low opinion of himself is confirmed, he drinks to relieve his guilt and shame
Refer the patient immediately to a psychiatrist	The patient does not keep his appoint-ment and continues drinking	Referral to a psychiatrist may be appropriate; however, drinking behavior must be interrupted for psychotherapy to help. Since alco-holics often drink to relieve de-pression, loneliness, and feelings of worthlessness, anything that makes the patient feel bad may increase his drinking. Abrupt referral to another doctor at this point may make the patient feel rejected and worthless, increasing the likelihood that he will drink. Also, since he has not agreed that he has a psychi-atric problem, he may see no reason to see a psychiatrist

A SUCCESSFUL APPROACH

Because the alcoholic is resistant to accepting his diagnosis and is humiliated by it, telling the patient that he is an alcoholic often involves some sort of confrontation. The doctor can reduce the inevitable embarrassment by remaining matter-of-fact and by communicating acceptance of the problem, concern for the patient's welfare, and hope for the possibility of change. Initial discussions have as their goal the patient's willingness to see that drinking may be causing problems in his life, rather than a confession that he is "alcoholic". This low-key approach is intended to circumvent the vicious circle of:

1. A strong confrontation makes the alcoholic feel hurt, rejected and embarrassed

2. He becomes angry and then feels guilty for being angry

3. He starts drinking to make himself feel better

4. He feels guilty for drinking, and drinks more to relieve this additional guilt

The following dialogue illustrates a useful approach:

Dr: Your tests show that you are drinking more than is good for you. No matter how much you are drinking, it's enough to be causing you some physical problems and to be affecting your work. Also, your wife is worried about your drinking. I'm asking you to join us so that we can discuss some ways for you to lick this problem. What do you think?

Pt: You may be right, but she'll just nag me.

Dr: Maybe we can help her to understand that you really aren't satisfied with how things have been going either, and come up with some ways she can be helpful to you.

Pt: You know, I'm not satisfied with my life. It seems
     like nothing interests me any more.

Dr: I'll bet you don't enjoy your hobbies either.

Pt: I guess you're right. I used to play golf and
     have woodworking projects. My wife and I don't
     even go to the movies now.

Dr: Drinking has a way of taking over people's lives
     without their realizing it. For example, did you
     change jobs voluntarily?

Pt: I lost my job after using up too much sick leave.

Dr: Your drinking caused you to take too much sick leave
     and I'm sure that made you feel even worse. I know
     you've had trouble keeping yourself from drinking
     when you feel bad. But with help from your wife
     and doctors, you should be able to make some progress.

The doctor has made a number of assumptions about the results of
the patient's drinking in order to bypass the patient's denial of his
problems while remaining firm in communicating his recommendations. It
also helps to:

1. Avoid arguing about the quantity of drinking or
    about the label of "alcoholic." Instead, emphasize
    that drinking has resulted in loss of job, interference
    with family life, or medical complications, even if
    the patient feels that he is in control of his drinking.

2. Involve the family. They can be helpful in identifying
    problems related to drinking and are crucial to
    effective treatment.

3. Convey to the patient that while the doctor is not
    going to go along with the patient's denial of his
    problem, he will not humiliate the patient by forcing
    him to admit to the mess he has made of his life. The
    patient will find it easier to deal with problems that
    have resulted from drinking if he does not fear being
    further exposed and embarrassed.

APPROACH TO OUTPATIENT MANAGEMENT

Diagnosing and treating a withdrawal syndrome is the first order of business with a hospitalized substance abuser. Next, the question of outpatient follow-up must be addressed. Once the patient feels a little better physically, he may become unrealistically optimistic and believe that he can get along without any further help, especially if admitting that he has a drinking problem would be a severe threat to his self-esteem. He then avoids feeling bad by denying the problem and feeling that there is no harm in using alcohol or other drugs again. If this occurs, the doctor should remain firm, while avoiding painful confrontations and continuing to emphasize the need to stop drinking.

The physician can follow the patient himself, especially if he has already established a positive relationship with the patient and his family. The support of a 10-15 minute chat about how it feels to be abstinent, and about physical, social, and emotional symptoms, can be extremely helpful. The patient should be given a return appointment one and three weeks after discharge, and monthly thereafter. The central nervous system probably requires at least 60 days to recover fully after withdrawal, and symptoms of irritability and emotional lability, in addition to the stresses of learning to live without drugs or alcohol, make the early months of abstinence especially difficult. Supportive follow-up is essential during this time and can be helpful indefinitely.

Taking drugs or drinking is almost reflexive whenever the abuser experiences unpleasant emotions. If he is not aware of this connection, he may find it difficult to understand the relapses that often occur. It is important that the doctor accept the patient's relapses in a non-judgmental manner and help him to identify the anger, depression or sense of failure or embarrassment that caused them, while conveying the hope that the patient will gradually improve.

Continued involvement of the family can be very helpful for ongoing identification of problems that precipitate increased drinking. The family also may need support themselves to understand the long-term nature of the patient's alcoholism. For example, they may attempt to enforce abstinence in a parental way, making the patient feel childish and increasing the likelihood he will drink. Such destructive inter-actions can be interrupted when the physician points them out and suggests alternative approaches.

The following dialogue illustrates some techniques that can be used in follow-up. The right-hand column comments on the patient's statements and the doctor's techniques:

Dialogue	*Comment*
Pt: Well, I haven't been drinking since you put me on Antabuse.	The patient places the responsibility for sobriety on the doctor. This is to be expected initially, and should not be confronted.
Dr: Have you missed drinking?	The doctor focuses the discussion on the patient's wish to drink.
Pt: I've been feeling better physically than I have in years, but I sure feel like having a drink when I get home at night.	The patient is able to recognize a reason of his own, not the doctor's, for not drinking (he feels better physically). However, he misses alcohol and feels tempted to drink.
Dr: Even though you feel better without drinking, it's tough to get along without alcohol after using it for so long.	Empathy with the patient offers support for the inevitable anxiety and depression that surface if the patient stops drowning them in alcohol. The doctor also indicates that drinking has been an important method of adaptation for the patient.
Pt: I even want a cocktail at lunch. Without it, I just feel like I can't get enough work done. The boss seems to think my work is fine, but I'm not satisfied with it.	The patient describes a perfectionistic attitude toward his work, which makes him anxious regardless of how well he is actually doing. Alcohol reduces this anxiety.
Dr: You seem to expect a lot of yourself.	The doctor now clarifies the patient's high expectations of himself. Later, he will help the patient to see how a perfectionistic attitude leads to a chronic sense of failure which the patient attempts to suppress with alcohol.

Treatment of substance abuse requires a long-term effort in which the following areas of the patient's thinking begin to change:

1. His perfectionism decreases, so that he can slowly stop denying his problem and begin to admit that he has human weaknesses, such as the need to depend on drugs or alcohol.

2. The patient's tendency to externalize the responsibility for treatment (and for his failures in life) slowly changes to a realization that he wants to be abstinent for his own sake, because it makes him feel better. He then is able to accept more responsibility for other aspects of his life.

3. As his denial decreases, he becomes aware of a struggle over whether to use drugs or not. This gradually evolves into acceptance of a drug-free life, as he learns to be comfortable with himself and to handle problems in ways that do not require drugs or alcohol.

The road to better functioning is a long one for substance abusers, as it is for many other physical and mental illnesses. The following guidelines are useful in this process.

1. Set regular appointments.

2. Keep an open-door policy. If the patient refuses follow-up, acknowledge the physician's awareness of the difficult problem he is facing. Indicate a willingness to keep working with his recurring problems in the hope that he will understand his difficulties better the next time.

3. Attempt to set a goal of long-term abstinence. There is currently no way of identifying in advance those few patients who will be able to resume normal drug or alcohol use without high risk of further abuse.

4. If the patient refuses to accept the goal of
    long-term abstinence, contract for a <u>trial</u>
    <u>period of abstinence</u> just to see how it works.
    Frequently, the patient is surprised at how
    good he feels and will be more open to the idea
    of long-term abstinence.

5. <u>Expect relapses</u>. By the time the substance abuser
    reaches treatment, his habit is firmly established,
    and more than one try may be required to break the
    pattern of abuse. An important part of the treatment
    plan is to continue to work with the patient during
    and after a relapse. Overcoming a substance abuse
    problem is much more difficult than dieting or
    stopping smoking, and the patient can be expected to
    revert to old habits under stress, at least early in
    treatment.

6. Use <u>Antabuse</u> unless it is contraindicated.

7. Feel free to make use of the following additional
    services:

    - <u>Specialized counseling</u> for alcohol and drug
      abusers is widely available through mental health
      centers and self-help groups. The psychiatric
      consultant can help to locate these programs.

    - <u>Alcoholics Anonymous</u> is available 24 hours a day
      and is as <u>successful</u> as any other treatment
      program (about two-thirds of patients improve).
      Have the patient call the number listed in the
      phone book while he is in the hospital. An A.A.
      member will visit.   A.A. offers support through
      fellowship and spiritual counseling as well as
      a detailed program for change through self-help.
      It works best for patients who:

        - are responsive to peers and social groups

        - are committed to abstinence and not just
          reduced drinking

        - are attracted by a spiritual approach

APPROACH TO MEDICATION

The substance abuser may have been using drugs for years as his only means of reducing emotional discomfort. It is therefore not surprising that many patients request a new medication after withdrawal. While it is best to avoid further use of drugs, the patient occasionally may need a prescription on a short-term basis until he can develop new ways of coping. If this is the case, it is helpful to tell the patient at the outset how long medication will be made available and to avoid prolonging whatever deadline is set.

Antabuse is a major exception. Because it is so difficult to give up a habit of long duration, Antabuse may be desirable to offer the alcoholic insurance against the temptation to drink. There are few reasons not to take this medication, and most patients should be offered a few months' trial. Antabuse reacts with alcohol to produce flushing, throbbing headache, respiratory difficulty, nausea, vomiting, sweating, and marked uneasiness. These symptoms should be described to the patient in detail, but he should not be given a trial experience of the alcohol-Antabuse reaction. Most patients do not drink on Antabuse if they understand what to expect. Antabuse primarily helps the patient to avoid impulsive drinking under stress, and some alcoholics discontinue the drug a few days before they anticipate needing a drink. Since a severe alcohol-Antabuse reaction can cause increased blood pressure and congestive heart failure, hypertension and cardiovascular disease are relative contraindications. However, the alcoholic is actually safer sober on Antabuse, since drinking also worsens hypertension and cardiovascular disease. Antabuse should not be given to a patient with an organic brain syndrome or psychosis severe enough to prevent his following the doctor's directions. Following are some guidelines for treatment with Antabuse:

1. Load the patient with 500 mg. of Antabuse
    daily for 5-7 days

2. Then give 250 mg. daily

3. Avoid daytime sedation by prescribing at bedtime

4. Treat rashes that occur occasionally with
    diphenhydramine (Benadryl) and by reducing the dose

5. Treat gastrointestinal distress (occurs occasionally) by reducing the dose

6. Remain alert to drug interactions:

   a. Increased effect of oral anticoagulants

   b. Increased blood levels of phenytoin

   c. Psychosis when administered with isoniazid and metronidazole

USE OF ADDICTIVE DRUGS

Doctors often are understandably reluctant to prescribe addictive drugs for substance abusers because of fear of further abuse. However, hospitalized patients frequently need sedative or analgesic medication in order to cope with their medical illness and with the psychological effects of hospitalization. The following points should be kept in mind, especially for opioids:

1. Prescribe adequate doses. Many physicians prescribe inadequate doses of narcotics, especially for hospitalized patients, because they are afraid of creating or continuing an addiction. However, continuing pain results in more of the patient's attention centering on pain and its relief, and more of his behavior becoming concerned with obtaining a narcotic. If the doctor does not argue with the patient about his medication, the chance of the patient's becoming addicted in the hospital is slight. Similarly, willingness to prescribe higher doses for a patient with a high tolerance for narcotics or a low pain threshold will not increase the chance of addiction and will make managing the patient easier.

2. Use a pharmacologically sound dosage schedule. Since the duration of action of many narcotics is 3-4 hours, most should be prescribed on a q 3h-q 4h schedule.

3. Offer the patient medication regularly (QID),
   q 4 hours, etc.) with the option to refuse.
   If a narcotic is offered PRN, the patient is
   forced to demonstrate pain in order to obtain
   medication. Offering him the option to refuse
   reduces the amount of begging or demanding in
   which he must engage to obtain relief and
   increases his confidence that pain will be
   relieved.

4. Increase the therapeutic effect of a drug by
   increasing its dose. If a medication does not
   produce a desired effect, increasing its dose
   or switching to another drug is less confusing
   than adding additional drugs in an attempt to
   achieve a synergistic effect.

5. Adjust the dosage depending on the route of
   administration. Most narcotics are more effective
   parenterally than orally, and the dose must be
   increased if the drug is given p.o.

6. Do not withdraw a patient when he is sick,
   especially if the medication to which he is
   addicted is appropriate in the management of
   his illness. Prescribe enough medication to
   prevent withdrawal and to achieve the needed
   sedative or analgesic effect until the illness
   is over, then begin withdrawal (if the patient
   agrees).

7. Do not attempt to withdraw a patient from a
   narcotic or sedative-hypnotic if he does not
   wish to be withdrawn. Even if the patient remains
   in the hospital long enough to complete withdrawal,
   he is likely to start medication again as soon as
   he is discharged.

8. Hospitalize a patient to withdraw him from an
   addicting drug. The temptation to continue taking
   the drug is usually too great for the patient
   to resist if its availability is not strictly
   controlled. Also, abstinence syndromes resulting
   from withdrawal of sedative-hypnotics and anti-anxiety
   drugs may be life-threatening. Patients who say that
   they wish to become drug-free but refuse hospitalization
   probably are not sufficiently motivated to withdraw
   anyway, no matter what rationalizations they offer.

9. Avoid starting a patient on a barbiturate,
    glutethimide (Doriden) or ethchlorvynol (Placidyl)
    for sleep. In the authors' experience, Flurazepam
    (Dalmane) and related compounds are less likely to
    interfere with normal sleep and to·produce severe
    physical dependence with its attendant abstinence
    syndrome and tendency toward addiction.

10. Follow guidelines and dosage schedules for the
    prescription of narcotics, tranquilizers, and
    sedative-hypnotics, and techniques for withdrawing
    patients from them, outlined in Tables 4.1-4.5
    (see pp. 137-147).

11. Remain alert for the following clues that a patient
    is exaggerating or falsifying symptoms in order to
    receive narcotics or is so untrustworthy that
    immediate psychiatric consultation is indicated for
    the management of a bona fide illness:

    a. Losing prescriptions or medications

    b. Repeatedly running out of medications
        before the time that would be expected
        if medications were taken as prescribed

    c. Obtaining narcotic or tranquilizer
        prescriptions from multiple physicians

    d. Claims that another doctor, who now cannot
        be located, prescribed a certain narcotic
        and that the patient now needs a refill

    e. Insistence on a particular strong narcotic
        (e.g. hydromorphone; Percodan) with the
        claim that nothing else will work

    f. Demands for the immediate prescription
        of a strong narcotic for a chronic illness

    g. Covert or overt threats when the physician
        does not comply with demands for narcotics

    h. Changing, dramatic descriptions of symptoms

    i. Any lying to the physician

12. Consider the use of a non-addicting nonsteroidal
     anti-inflammatory drug. Zomepirac (Zomax),
     50-100 mg. q 4-6h, or ibuprofen (Motrin)
     400 mg. q 4-6h, are effective for mild to moderate
     pain, although they do not control severe pain.

PROGNOSIS

The misconception that prognosis is poor in substance abuse
frequently makes it difficult for many physicians to feel optimistic
about treating substance abusers, especially alcoholics. This negative
view comes in part from exposure in medical school to "end - stage"
alcoholics. In fact, fewer than 5% of alcoholics are in "skid row",
and only 1% have cirrhosis. Studies of outcomes of a wide variety of
therapies demonstrate that of alcoholics in treatment:

     - one-third will remain sober for years

     - one-third will do well for a year or so and
       then drink again

     - one-third will continue drinking

Thus, two-thirds of alcoholics can be expected to improve. If
this hopeful attitude is transmitted to the patient, his sense of
support and acceptance as he struggles with his problem increases.

DIFFERENTIAL DIAGNOSIS

In 25-30% of substance abusers the abuse problem is secondary to
another disorder, in which the patient drinks or takes drugs in an
attempt to treat the underlying problem. Conditions commonly confused
with primary substance abuse are considered below, along with salient
differentiating features:

Psychiatric Diagnosis	_Salient Differentiating Features_
Patients may attempt to reduce feelings of <u>depression</u> by drinking or taking drugs. The incidence of suicide attempts is significantly higher in the intoxicated state, when inhibitions to impulsive behavior are decreased. Since alcohol or drug abuse is not an effective treatment, the underlying depression does not improve and substance abuse continues	- Vegetative signs (e.g., sleep disturbance, diurnal variation, appetite disturbance, weight change) are present in depression - Depressive feelings antedated the onset of substance abuse - Depression worsens when the patient stops drinking
Self-limited <u>depressive symptoms</u> often are seen in the early months after <u>withdrawal</u>, as a normal reaction to the changes in the patient's life and to his increasing realization of the problems his substance abuse has created	- Depressive symptoms decrease within a few months - Vegetative signs are absent
Some patients with <u>incipient psychoses</u> attempt to prevent psychotic decompensation with large amounts of alcohol or drugs. The appearance of psychotic symptoms when they stop the drug may be mistaken for an abstinence syndrome	- Hallucinations are usually auditory - Thought disorder (loose associations, etc.) is present on close examination - Obvious signs of schizophrenia or other psychosis appear on drug withdrawal

Psychiatric Diagnosis	*Salient Differentiating Features*
In patients with borderline or explosive personality disorders, abuse of alcohol or drugs is secondary to a characterologic inability to tolerate feelings and impulses and is one of a number of symptoms of major maladjustment	- Life-long maladaptive pattern of handling stress - Excitable, hostile, aggressive and impulsive behavior is evident when the patient is drug free - Poor interpersonal relationships - Lack of a clear sense of identity
The patient with an antisocial personality disorder has repeated conflicts with the law and shallow, self-serving relationships with other people and with society. Substance abuse, especially involving stealing and selling drugs, is common in these patients as one of a number of anti-social behaviors	- Chronic, repetitive, conflict with the law, beginning in adolescence - No allegiance to individuals, groups, or social values - Lack of guilt or shame - Inability to learn from experience or punishment

USE OF THE PSYCHIATRIST

The primary physician should consult with a psychiatrist to:

1. Develop a treatment plan

2. Decide whether to withdraw the patient from opiates, tranquilizers, or sedative-hypnotics

3. Obtain help in arranging for follow-up by a specialized agency

4. Discuss his own reaction and that of his staff to the patient

5. Differentiate between substance abuse and
    other psychiatric disorders

6. Understand the significance of lying,
    about drug use

7. Determine how to proceed with an addict who
    needs analgesics or sedatives

The physician should <u>refer the patient to a psychiatrist</u>
when:

1. The patient expresses an interest in psychiatric
    treatment

2. The patient has an unusual degree of anxiety
    or depression

3. The patient has psychotic symptoms after
    withdrawal

4. Marked antisocial features are present

5. The physician does not wish to prescribe narcotics
    or tranquilizers for a substance abuser

Table 4.1

INTOXICATION AND WITHDRAWAL FROM ABUSED SUBSTANCES AND METHODS OF DETOXIFICATION

Drug	Symptoms of Intoxication	Withdrawal Syndrome	Method of Detoxification
HALLUCINOGENS, e.g., LSD, mescaline – peyote, marijuana	Flushing of skin, dilated pupils, transient increases in pulse rate and blood pressure, auditory and visual hallucinations, marked anxiety, depression, suicidal thoughts, confusion, paranoid ideation	None	None required. "Bad trips" can be treated with diazepam (Valium) or, more simply, by "talking down" through verbal reassurance and emotional support
ARYLCYCLOHEXAMINES, e.g., phencylidine (PCP), ketamine	Anxiety, agitation, violence, euphoria, nystagmus ataxia, dysarthria, diaphoresis, hypertension	None	Minimize social stimulation and place in quiet room. Avoid tranquilizers
STIMULANTS, e.g., amphetamines, cocaine, Tenuate, Preludin, Ritalin	Restlessness, irritability, anxiety, tachycardia, dry mouth, cardiac arrhythmia, acute OBS, paranoid psychosis with clear sensorium	Mild to moderate depression with fatigue and somatic complaints for several weeks. In some cases, the patient may "crash" with severe depression and suicidal ideation	None required usually. Psychiatric hospitalization for severe symptoms

Table 4.1 contd.

Drug	Symptoms of Intoxication	Withdrawal Syndrome	Method of Detoxification
OPIOIDS, e.g., heroin, morphine, Dilaudid, Demerol, Percodan, codeine	Miosis, euphoria, drowsiness	Moderate flu-like symptoms beginning in first 24 hours and lasting 3-5 days	Can be accomplished "cold turkey" or with antianxiety agents, methadone or clonidine. (Details in Table 4.5)
SEDATIVE-HYPNOTICS, e.g., barbiturates, chloral hydrate, Doriden, Noludar, Quaalude, Placidyl	Mental impairment, confusion, nystagmus, motor incoordination, ataxia, depression, dysarthria, postural hypotension	Weakness, insomnia, nausea, and postural hypotension develop in the first 48 hours and last 5-7 days. Seizures may occur at any time, especially in the first few days. Delirium may develop between the 3rd and 7th day and lasts 3-5 days	See Table 4.4
ANTI-ANXIETY AGENTS, e.g., Librium, Valium, Serax, Tranxene, Verstran, meprobamate, Dalmane, Restoril, Ativan	Symptoms are similar to those seen with sedative-hypnotics, but milder	Prolonged, attenuated symptoms, chiefly anxiety, may last 7-10 days. Seizures may occur with withdrawal from meprobamate or high doses of benzodiazepines (more than 40-60 mg/day of diazepam or equivalent)	If symptoms are severe, proceed as for sedative-hypnotics

Table 4.1 contd.

Drug	Symptoms of Intoxication	Withdrawal Syndrome	Method of Detoxification
ALCOHOL	Mental impairment, confusion, motor incoordination, ataxia, aggressiveness, release of inhibitions	Four syndromes are seen: the shakes, withdrawal seizures, delirium tremens, and hallucinosis/paranoia (See Table 4.2)	Simple cases of the shakes can be handled on an outpatient basis or in a non-medical 24 hour care setting; otherwise, hospitalization is required (See Table 4.2)

Table 4.2

ALCOHOL WITHDRAWAL

Syndrome	Detoxification
The Shakes - tachycardia, tremulousness, sweating, nausea, beginning within first 24 hours and lasting 3-4 days	Chlorazepate (Tranxene) 60 mg. on the 1st day, 30 mg. on the 2nd day, 15 mg. on the 3rd day, then discontinue. Thiamine 100 mg. i.m. q day for 3 days
Withdrawal Seizures - 1 or 2 grand mal seizures may occur in the first 48 hours in less than 1% of untreated cases of the shakes	Add diazepam (Valium) 10 mg. i.m. or i.v. on the first day to medication for the shakes. Dilantin is not needed for withdrawal seizures unless the patient is an epileptic
Delirium Tremens - tachycardia, fever, confusion, psychosis, and gross shaking begin after 72 hours and may be preceded by a withdrawal seizure. Lasts 5-7 days. Occurs in 1% or less of cases of the shakes. Episodes of D.T.'s that are uncomplicated by other medical problems (e.g., pancreatitis, subdural hematoma) are not fatal	Chlordiazepoxide (Librium) 50-100 mg. i.m. QID or until sedated. Add Haloperidol (Haldol) 5 mg. i.m. q 4 hr. prn agitation, hallucinations, delusions. Thiamine 100 mg. q D. for 3-4 days. Keep an intravenous line open and taper medications over 4 days.
Hallucinosis/Paranoia - hallucinations or delusions without gross confusion may begin while the patient is still drinking or during withdrawal. May last up to several weeks but rarely becomes chronic. Occurs in 0.5% of cases of the shakes.	Haloperidol 10-30 mg. per day

Table 4.3

PRESCRIBING ADDICTIVE DRUGS

Generic Name	Proprietary Name	Usual Dose	Indications	Comments
NARCOTICS: Morphine Hydromorphine Meperidine	Dilaudid Demerol	10 mg. q 4 hr. 1.5-2 mg. q 4 hr. 50-100 mg. q 2-4 hr.	-Analgesia	Only 1/5-1/4 of orally administered doses of morphine, hydromorphine, and meperidine are absorbed
Pentazocine	Talwin	50 mg. po or 30 mg. im q 4 hr.		-Has agonist and antagonist properties, and will nullify analgesic effect of other narcotics if given concomitantly
Oxycodone	Percodan	5 mg. po q 4 hr.		-High addictive potential
Codeine		30 mg. q 4 hr.		-Low addictive potential
Propoxyphene	Darvon	65 mg. q 4 hr.		-Addictive, but no more effective than aspirin or acetaminophen
Methadone	Dolophine	5-10 mg. q 3-5 hr.		-Effective in the treatment of chronic pain while producing less euphoria

Table 4.3 contd.

Generic Name	Proprietary Name	Usual Dose	Indications	Comments
BENZODIAZEPINES:				
Diazepam	Valium	5 mg. QID	-Temporary anxiety	-Mild side effects--typically hangover, dizziness
Chlordiaze- poxide	Librium	10 mg. QID	-Muscle relaxation	-Dependence begins at 4-5 times the normal dose for 2-3
Oxazepam	Serax	10 mg. QID	-Valium also for acute	months, and is not as common as was once feared
Chlorazepate	Tranxene	7.5 mg. QID	seizure control	-Long half-life may allow single daily dose
Lorazepam	Ativan	1 mg. QID	-May be used to potentiate analgesics	-Potentiate CNS depressant drugs including alcohol
				-Very safe--overdose not lethal
				-Poorly absorbed when adminis- tered intramuscularly
				-Blood levels are increased by concomitantly administered cimetidine
Flurazepam	Dalmane	30 mg. qhs	-Insomnia	-Does not depress REM sleep
Temazepam	Restoril	30 mg. qhs		-A new hypnotic with perhaps a shorter half-life than Flurazepam

Table 4.3 contd.

Generic Name	Proprietary Name	Usual Dose	Indications	Comments
BARBITURATES, RELATED COMPOUNDS:				
Amobarbital	Amytal	100 mg. qhs	-Insomnia	-Side effects - hangover, dizziness, ataxia
Secobarbital	Seconal	100 mg. qhs	-Phenobarbital also for seizure control	-More addictive than benzodiazepines
Pentobarbital	Nembutal	100 mg. qhs		-Tolerance common
Phenobarbital	Luminal	130 mg. qhs		-Withdrawal symptoms severe
Methaqualone	Quaalude	150 mg. qhs		-Potentiate CNS depressants
				-Narrow range of safety; overdoses often lethal
				-Paradoxical excitement may be seen
				-Phenobarbital decreases blood levels of many other drugs
Glutethimide	Doriden	500 mg. qhs	-Rarely used for insomnia	-Because these drugs interfere with normal sleep, are frequently abused, are extremely dangerous when taken in overdose and produce prolonged abstinence syndromes, they are poor choices as hypnotics
Ethchlorvynol	Placidyl	500 mg. qhs		

Table 4.3 contd.

Generic Name	Proprietary Name	Usual Dose	Indications	Comments
Meprobamate	Equanil	400 mg. QID	-Temporary anxiety -Muscle relaxation	-High abuse potential -Medical management of over-dose is difficult
CHLORAL COMPOUNDS:				
Chloral-hydrate	Noctec	500 mg. hs	-Insomnia	-A good choice if flurazepam, temazepam and antihistamines are ineffective

Table 4.4

WITHDRAWAL TECHNIQUE FOR ANY COMBINATION OF
SLEEPING PILLS, ANTI-ANXIETY AGENTS AND ALCOHOL

1. Because of the danger of seizures and delirium, and of the
    likelihood that outpatients will continue to take medications
    or drink, withdrawal should only be attempted in the hospital.

2. Do not believe what the patient says about how much he takes.
    Instead, estimate the degree of tolerance to these cross-
    tolerant drugs by administering 200 mg. of pentobarbital p.o.,
    preferably on an empty stomach, and observe one hour later
    for signs of intoxication (positive Romberg, ataxia, finger-
    to-nose incoordination, nystagmus, slurred speech, drowsiness,
    postural hypotension). Then:

    a. Prevent precipitous withdrawal by giving
        pentobarbital in doses predicted by the
        test in 2, above:

        - No Tolerance: drowsy or asleep when
          tested - no medication required.

        - Moderate Tolerance: moderate symptoms.
          Give 200-300 mg. pentobarbital p.o. q
          6 hours or 60-90 mg. phenobarbital p.o.
          q 6 hours.

        - Extreme Tolerance: few or no symptoms.
          Give 400-500 mg. pentobarbital p.o. q 6
          hours or 150-180 mg. phenobarbital p.o.
          q 6 hours.

    b. Adjust the initial dose so that no symptoms
        of withdrawal are seen.

    c. Reduce the dose by 10% every 1-2 days, watching
        for symptoms of either withdrawal or intoxication
        as a guide to the speed of reduction. When
        pentobarbital is administered, seizures may
        occur if any dose is administered late.

Table 4.4 contd.

3. The physician also may use a test dose of 60-100 mg. of
    phenobarbital p.o. or i.m. Subsequent 60 mg. doses are
    given every 2-6 hours until symptoms of intoxication
    appear. The total dose of phenobarbital required to
    produce intoxication is then given daily in 4 evenly
    divided doses, and withdrawn as in c, above.

4. Because phenobarbital has a long half-life that may lead
    to excessive accumulation when high doses are administered
    for more than a few days, some clinicians administer 60-90
    mg. of phenobarbital q6h for 2 days in cases of moderate,
    uncomplicated withdrawal and then discontinue. Others
    simply reduce the dose more rapidly if intoxication appears.

Table 4.5

OPIOID WITHDRAWAL TECHNIQUES

1. Because of the difficulty of ensuring that the patient
    will not obtain medication if his environment is not
    controlled, withdrawal is best accomplished in the
    hospital

2. Do not believe what the patient says about how much he
    takes. Instead, in the presence of manifest withdrawal
    symptoms, start the patient on 30 mg. methadone p.o.
    daily

3. Adjust the dose to prevent withdrawal symptoms, up to
    50 mg. of methadone daily

4. Taper off of methadone by reducing the dose by 10%
    per day

5. The physician also may abruptly discontinue the narcotic
    and use anti-anxiety drugs to suppress withdrawal symptoms

6. Clonidine hydrochloride, 0.1-0.3 mg. PO TID for 2 weeks
    also ameliorates symptoms of opiate withdrawal. Blood
    pressure should be monitored closely and the drug should
    be tapered during the last few days of treatment

REFERENCES

American Medical Association: <u>Manual on Alcoholism</u>. Chicago,
    American Medical Association, 1970.

Ewing, JA, Blakewell WE: ˙Diagnosis and Reaction of Drug
    Dependence of the Barbiturate Type. <u>Amer J Psychiatry</u>
    1968; 125:6.

Frosch WA: Narcotic Addiction   In: <u>Current Therapy</u>.
    Philadelphia, WB Saunders, 1973.

Gessner PK: Drug Therapy of the Alcohol Withdrawal Syndrome.
    In <u>Biochemistry and Pharmacology of Ethanol</u>, Vol. 2,
    Plenum, 1979.

Gold MS, Pottash AC, Sweeney DR, Kleber HD: Opiate Withdrawal
    Using Clonidine. <u>JAMA</u> 1980; 243:343.

Chapter Six
REACTIONS TO ILLNESS

When a person becomes ill, he must come to terms not only with physical discomfort but with the special significance being sick may hold for him. For one thing, every illness can create a loss of function, income, security, independence or even life. If the patient is hospitalized, he also must endure separation from loved ones that can be particularly difficult if the patient is dependent on his family, or afraid that they will desert him. Illness also involves loss of control over the patient's body, his future, and, for the inpatient, over everyday decisions, for example about when to eat and when to sleep. Every patient also must face the need to depend on physicians and nurses at least temporarily, as well as on family members for as long as he is ill.

Past experiences with illness and caretaking affect reactions to illness in the present. Patients who have learned that people who take care of them can be relied upon to protect and not abandon them and that being sick is not a devastating experience usually accept the need to depend on others, relinquish control to them gracefully, and tolerate loss of function and separation from loved ones well, especially when they know that these are temporary. However, patients whose parents or other caretakers were unreliable, became angry when they were ill or otherwise did not allow them to become comfortable with normal dependency may feel that present-day parental figures (e.g., physicians) will prove as untrustworthy as those in the past. This and other concerns may arouse anxiety that leads to a number of maladaptive behaviors (described below).

The enforced passivity and dependence that accompany illness and its treatment may encourage a return to a level of psychological development appropriate to a time in the patient's life when he was more dependent, i.e., childhood. This regression also relieves anxiety about dependency and loss of control, since a child has fewer conflicts about these issues. It manifests itself as child-like, demanding, complaining behavior and low frustration tolerance, and often is puzzling and disturbing to both physician and patient.

In order to keep anxiety that is aroused by being sick and/or hospitalized at tolerable levels, patients may attempt to deny (ignore) or minimize the seriousness of their condition. Denial, like other ego defenses that keep anxiety within tolerable limits, often serves a useful function. For example, if the physician always empathized totally with his patients' fear, suffering and despair, he would be so distracted by his emotional reaction that it would be impossible to care for them effectively. Similarly, if the patient who has suffered a recent myocardial infarction were overwhelmed with anxiety about his prospects for recovery, he might not only find it difficult to accept necessary treatment passively, but excess catecholamine secretion might adversely affect his heart. It is only when defenses are so rigid that they interfere with, rather than promote, adaptation (e.g., by interfering with the physician's ability to empathize with the patient at all or by preventing the patient from complying with therapy) that coping ability is reduced.

If attempts to control anxiety by denying the severity of the illness are unsuccessful, the patient may deny awareness of the illness itself. Consider, for example, the 48-year-old physician who develops crushing substernal chest pain. He realizes immediately that he may be having a myocardial infarction and is extremely frightened. He relaxes as he convinces himself that he is really just suffering from heartburn, and his wife must finally demand that he seek medical attention. Such denial can result in a 4-5 hour delay after developing severe pain of myocardial infarction before most patients seek medical attention and probably contributes to the enormous mortality rate (about 60% of coronary deaths) in myocardial infarction patients before they reach the hospital.

When a patient seeks medical assistance, his doctor confers the sick role on him. The patient agrees to seek help, follow orders, accept dependency, and try to get well. In return, he is exempted from his normal responsibilities. The patient leaves the sick role by being pronounced cured by the doctor, by refusing further treatment, or by dying. While many people are able to tolerate the sick role, and some seek it (e.g., the hypochondriacal patient), others may have great difficulty accepting care, taking orders, or giving up the responsibilities of the "healthy role," even temporarily. Refusal to participate in treatment may indicate that the patient is finding it difficult to accept some aspect of the sick role.

Reactions to the patient's illness occur in the patient's family, too. They may not understand the patient's illness. The disorganization of normal family life and role reversal that are caused by the illness may manifest themselves as confusion as to what is really wrong with the patient. Family members also may be afraid of separation from the patient, resulting in a fear that the patient will die, even if he is in no danger. Numerous other feelings, described in chapter **7**, may interfere with the patient's ability to adapt to his illness.

Physicians and nurses also cannot help reacting to the patient's illness. They may put themselves in the patient's place (identify with him) and experience the patient's emotions, or those feelings they would experience if they were sick themselves. More commonly, however, they attempt to avoid such emotions by distancing themselves from the patient through aloofness, lack of understanding of the patient, or anger at him. Understanding and dealing with these reactions is essential to successful patient management. It may also happen that the physician or nursing staff's reaction is conditioned by factors not directly related to the patient. For example, if a house officer has been criticized excessively by his attending physician, he may find himself losing his temper with his patients. Or a physician who has experienced a death in his family may feel either overly pessimistic or optimistic with a dying patient who reminds him of his relative. While the source of the doctor's reaction may be obvious to an unbiased observer, it may not be at all obvious to the physician or his staff.

Despite the emotional crisis that may be caused by an acute illness, the patient at least can be reassured that his condition will reverse itself. The chronically ill patient, on the other hand, must face life without any hope of a cure. Concerns about being sick then are greatly intensified, several worries being particularly common. First, fears of a permanent loss of income become quite realistic, and significant readjustments in lifestyle may be necessary, as is acceptance of permanent limitations in the patient's goals for himself. The patient also must come to terms with a more or less permanent loss of control over a major part of his life: Even though treatment may prevent further decompensation, no matter how hard the patient tries he cannot make himself better. As a result, some patients may ignore medical advice on the grounds that it will not cure them anyway, while others may actively worsen their illnesses in order to feel some sense of control. Many self-destructive forms of noncompliance seen in chronically ill patients (e.g., the diabetic who neglects his insulin or the dialysis patient who ignores dietary restrictions) are motivated by a feeling of helplessness and an attempt to regain at least the illusion of control over one's illness.

Chronic illness also has a profound effect on families. Just as the patient may find it difficult to relinquish the role of caretaker and provider, the spouse and children may wish to continue being more dependent on the patient than is possible. Sexual dysfunction is created by many chronic illnesses and their treatments, and the physician also must evaluate the family's ability to grieve lost functions and roles. A major goal is to avoid divorce, a regrettably common means of avoiding the painful tasks that confront the chronically ill.

Reactions of patients, their families, and their physicians are intensified in the case of terminal illnesses, where universal concerns about separation, helplessness, and death are aroused. The management of the dying patient, and of grief reactions in the survivors, are discussed later in this chapter, after denial, noncompliance and regression have been considered.

DENIAL

ENCOUNTER WITH A TYPICAL PATIENT

Mrs. R., a previously healthy, 32-year-old mother of two, developed fatigue and easy bruising a month ago. She ascribed her symptoms to being "run down" and did not consult a doctor until her husband noticed that she looked very pale and insisted that she be examined. She was found to be anemic and was admitted for further workup.

On examination she is pale and haggard, with bruises on her forearms and thighs. Initial hemoglobin is 9, platelet count 35,000, and white blood count 60,000.

On the second hospital day the physician discusses with Mrs. R. the tests he would like to order. When she seems reluctant to agree to a bone marrow aspiration, he explains its importance in making a diagnosis. The following conversation then ensues:

Pt: I've been feeling better since I got here--maybe I don't need the test.

Dr: I'm happy that you're feeling better, but I still feel that we must find out what's wrong with you.

Pt: Maybe nothing is seriously wrong.

Dr: I hope so. However, your blood tests are abnormal, and we do need to rule out a number of diseases.

Pt: I don't like to disagree, but I don't think I need any more tests right now.

THE PHYSICIAN'S REACTION TO HIS PATIENT

If the doctor is preoccupied by his own feelings about the patient, he will find it difficult to listen to and understand the patient's reaction to his illness. Following are some common emotions physicians feel after the kind of interaction just described, along with comments on their significance.

Physician's Reaction	*Comment*
Anger with the patient	It is natural to become angry when the patient rejects the doctor's efforts to be helpful and does not seem to find his opinion important. Anger also can serve to distance the doctor from the patient, lessening the impact on him of a terrible illness affecting a woman who is not far from his own age
Feeling that there is nothing that can be done to help the patient	Many physicians feel helpless when a patient does not respond to interventions that usually are effective. This reaction also may reflect the doctor's feeling about the patient having a potentially fatal illness
Not minding if the patient signed out of the hospital	If the doctor feels angry and helpless, he may wish to decrease his discomfort by distancing himself emotionally from the patient. This may even take the form of covert encouragement to leave the hospital, e.g., by refusing to listen to the patient's objections to a test or procedure or generally becoming less sensitive to her feelings

Physician's Reaction	*Comment*
Wish to resolve the physician's confusion about why the patient will not cooperate by talking some sense into her	The patient's reaction is confusing. Many people respond to ambiguity by doing more of what they already know how to do. The physician who feels most comfortable in an authoritarian role therefore may act more authoritarian when he is unsure as to how to proceed

COMMON UNSUCCESSFUL APPROACHES

When physicians are confronted by a patient's denial of the seriousness of his illness, they may apply one of several approaches. These are listed below, opposite the patient's response and an explanation of the patient's behavior.

Physician's Approach	*Patient's Response*	*Explanation*
Try harder to convince the patient that she is sick	The patient insists more strenuously that she is healthy	The patient is frightened by the possibility of being seriously ill. She attempts to ignore (deny) her fear by denying that there is anything to worry about. When the doctor insists that she is sick she becomes more anxious. Since the only defense available at this time is denial, her denial increases, too

Physician's Approach	Patient's Response	Explanation
Tell the patient that if she does not agree to more tests she may die of leukemia	The patient leaves the hospital immediately	The patient's anxiety increases greatly in response to this suggestion. If the amount of anxiety exceeds the patient's psychological capacity to deny, she may take physical action to avoid the situation (being in the hospital) that makes her anxious
Tell the patient that she is reacting abnormally to the possibility of being sick	The patient does not understand what the doctor is talking about	Since the patient's denial occurs automatically, she is unlikely to be aware of it even if it is pointed out, and may deny this insight as well as other information

A SUCCESSFUL APPROACH

If a patient uses excessive denial to control anxiety, approaches aimed at making her aware of her fear are likely to increase denial and refusal to cooperate. However, agreeing with the patient that she is not sick does her a disservice. The doctor must instead find a way to decrease the patient's anxiety without immediately confronting the issue that frightens her:

Dr: I'd like you to stay in the hospital a while longer for a few more tests.

Pt: I don't see why--I'm feeling better.

Dr: It's good that you're feeling better, and there may well be nothing to worry about. But I'd feel better if you'd just stay for the tests.

Pt: But if there's nothing wrong, why do I need to stay?

Dr: It will help me to get a more complete.picture of your
     state of health so I can treat you better.

Pt: But maybe I don't need treatment.

Dr: That may be. But as your doctor I'll still need to
     keep in touch with you, and I'd 'feel better about doing
     so if I can get the tests done.

Pt: Well, if it will help you, I suppose I could stay,
     if it's not such a big deal.

The doctor has shifted the focus of concern to himself without
affirming or denying that he thinks that the patient is sick. At the
same time he is firm in his request that she stay without being so
authoritarian that the patient is provoked into arguing with him.
Instead, the patient may "save face" because she is staying to please
the doctor.

THE PATIENT WHO THREATENS TO SIGN OUT AGAINST MEDICAL ADVICE

Occasionally, a patient with an acute life-threatening illness
escalates denial as the danger he faces becomes more obvious and he
feels less equipped to control anxiety in any other way. The patient
may then insist that since he is not sick, he does not need to be in the
hospital, despite obvious evidence of serious pathology. The patient
politely listens to the doctor's arguments that he may die if he leaves,
and then insists even more strenuously that he plans to sign out. This
situation is most likely to arise in patients with acute medical illnesses (e.g., an acute M.I. patient who insists on leaving after his
first day on the C.C.U.), or in patients requiring surgery for correction
of life-threatening conditions (e.g., the patient with abdominal pain
who refuses appendectomy). Such extreme denial is most likely to occur
after the pain that brought the patient to the hospital subsides enough
for him to ignore it.

If the approach to acute denial described above is unsuccessful,
and the patient's life would be in danger if he left the hospital, the
following additional steps may be useful in managing this situation:

1. Do not spend a great deal of time attempting to convince
    the patient that he is sick. Simply tell him that it is
    important that he remain in the hospital for a few days
    more. If he argues that he is not ill, tell him that
    his physician wants him to stay, whether or not he feels
    sick.

2. If the patient assumes a self-important air and insists
    that no young doctor is going to tell him what to do, the
    chief of service or most senior physician available should
    tell the patient, in an authoritative manner, that he must
    remain in the hospital.

3. Encourage the patient to ventilate his feelings about
    ward care, and correct realistic problems that have
    arisen.

4. If family members of friends are available, explain the
    seriousness of the situation to them and ask them to
    convince the patient to cooperate. If they are not
    readily available, ask the patient to stay until they
    can be located.

5. Consider bargaining with the patient around treatment
    issues, conceding certain requirements in return for the
    patient's promise to remain hospitalized.

6. If the patient still refuses to stay, and his illness
    is so dangerous that death or serious disability would
    result from his signing out, a temporary "mental health
    hold" may be obtained to keep him in the hospital on the
    grounds that the patient is a danger to himself. In many
    states, a "mental illness" (e.g., depression) also must be
    said to be present. The hold may be signed by any
    physician in most states. Time spent equivocating once
    it is clear the patient plans to leave usually is wasted,
    and the patient often is relieved to have the doctor take
    over the responsibility for the decision to stay. Severe
    denial is likely to resolve over a few days and most
    patients decide to stay voluntarily. While it is a good
    idea to consult with an attorney before proceeding with a
    mental health hold, the danger to the patient's life often
    outweighs the threat of legal retribution (which is rare)
    once the patient has recovered.

DETERMINATION OF COMPETENCY

While the physician must take responsibility for making life and death decisions for patients whose lives are in immediate danger, others must be permitted to refuse treatment even though their lives may eventually be forfeit. Competency to refuse or to consent to medical therapy is said to be present when the patient understands:

1.   The nature of his illness

2.   The potential benefits of treatment and its mechanism of action

3.   The consequences of refusing treatment

Even the psychotic patient who understands his illness, the treatment, and the consequences of refusing therapy is legally competent to refuse medical care.

The following guidelines apply when a patient does not wish to consent to needed treatment:

1.   If the patient is in dire need of treatment and cannot or will not consent to treatment, the physician should act to keep the patient alive as described above. The physician should document the need for immediate care and obtain consent from a family member if possible.

2.   A mental status examination (see pp. 86-91) should be performed if an organic brain syndrome may be interfering with the patient's ability to understand and consent to medical care.

3.   The competent patient who is not in danger of dying immediately of an acute condition cannot be required to undergo treatment against his will, even if refusal ultimately will result in his death. This is the case for many patients who refuse needed maintenance therapy such as dialysis.

NONCOMPLIANCE

Failure to follow therapeutic regimens is probably more common than meticulous compliance with the doctor's orders. At least 15% and as many as 93% of medical outpatients are noncompliant at some point during their treatment, either failing to follow the treatment plan at all, complying intermittently, and/or adding idiosyncratic remedies. A wish to deny that one is sick enough to require treatment is one reason why noncompliance occurs. Other factors include:

1. Absence of pain or other symptoms or disability that appear soon after the drug is discontinued. If the nature of the illness is such that the patient does not feel uncomfortable as soon as he stops the drug (e.g., hypertension, epilepsy), the patient may not feel that he really needs it.

2. Difficulty following a complicated regimen. Patients who must take a number of different pills many times each day may confuse medications with each other, fail to keep track of which pills have been taken, or feel overwhelmed and only take some of the prescribed drugs.

3. Reluctance to trust the physician and his therapy. The patient may not have faith in the physician because he does not know the doctor well, thinks that the clinician does not like him, is generally suspicious, distrusts authority figures, or is from a cultural background that offers explanations of the illness and its treatment that differ from the physician's.

4. Belief that, since a chronic illness cannot be cured, it is pointless to invest oneself in treatments that at best only slow down its progression.

5. Belief that the treatment is unnecessary or useless, either because symptoms have abated (e.g., partially treated infections) or the drug has a delayed onset of action (e.g., antidepressants).

6. Hopelessness about the possibility of a cure. Depressed patients, especially those with severe depressions, may feel that since they will never improve no matter what they do, antidepressants or other treatments will be of no use. Some depressed patients also may not follow the treatment regimen because they feel that they do not deserve to improve.

7. Self-destructive wishes, expressed as a desire to die of the illness or to suffer when it is not cured.

8. Failure on the physician's part to convey sufficient confidence that treatment will be effective.

9. Inability to afford medication, follow-up visits or adjunctive treatments.

10. Fear of side effects, e.g., of the impotence that may be caused by antihypertensive drugs. Exaggerated fears of side effects may result from the physician's over-enthusiastic description in great detail of rare but dangerous or upsetting actions in a wish to inform the patient fully, or from warnings from friends who have had untoward experiences with the treatment.

11. Inability to remember the treatment plan or medications that have been taken. Demented patients are particularly likely to have this problem.

12. Wish to frustrate the physician. Some chronically unhappy people take out their frustration on the physician by subtly thwarting his attempts to be helpful. They then feel some sense of control in making the physician feel as frustrated and unhappy as they feel.

THE PHYSICIAN'S REACTION TO THE NONCOMPLIANT PATIENT

It is difficult to avoid feeling angry with a patient who ignores one's advice and thwarts one's attempts to be helpful, particularly when the patient says that he is following the treatment plan but is discovered to be covertly noncompliant. In addition, physicians often feel helpless to influence noncompliant patients positively, or become convinced that the patient must be mentally ill to refuse to adhere to a rational treatment. Some clinicians also may feel that they will be held responsible for the patient's failure to improve.

COMMON UNSUCCESSFUL APPROACHES

Several commonly applied approaches to the noncompliant patient are described below, along with the patient's response and the reasons why the patient responds as he does.

Physician's Approach	*Patient's Response*	*Explanation*
Attempt to frighten the patient into complying by telling him that he will die if he does not take medication as prescribed	The patient says that he will comply but does not	Denial of the need for medication is a prominent mechanism of noncompliance. Attempts to overcome denial and force the patient to see the truth usually result in an increase in denial as the patient attempts to protect himself from information he finds threatening
Wait for the patient's condition to worsen so that he may learn what a mistake it is not to comply	The patient's noncompliance continues until he becomes dangerously ill. He then accepts hospital treatment but is noncompliant again after discharge	The noncompliant patient already is able to ignore the fact that compliance is in his best interest. There is little reason to expect this behavior to change until the reasons for its occurrence, which follow the patient's inner logic rather than external reality, can be elucidated and dealt with

Physician's Approach	*Patient's Response*	*Explanation*
Spend more time with the patient in an effort to convey the physician's interest in seeing him improve	The patient is happy to see the physician and seems cooperative at each visit. However, due to continuing noncompliance he requires more intensive follow-up	As the patient learns that he can gain the physician's interest and attention by remaining ill, he continues his covert efforts at undoing attempts at a cure, which would result in his seeing less, rather than more, of the physician

A SUCCESSFUL APPROACH

Enhancing compliance depends on the physician's ability to establish a trusting relationship with the patient, address in advance situations that are likely to be associated with noncompliance, discuss noncompliance in an open but nonthreatening manner, and help the patient to find other means of dealing with the concerns that lead him to omit his medication according to the following guidelines:

1. Explain the treatment plan in simple non-technical language. When a complex regimen is required, ask the patient to repeat instructions back to the physician.

2. Convey appropriate confidence in the therapeutic regimen. The patient may find it particularly difficult to adhere to a treatment plan in which the doctor does not seem to have much faith.

3. Make sure that the patient can afford the treatment. This obvious issue may be overlooked by the busy physician who assumes that the patient would not accept a prescription he could not afford.

4. Prescribe as few pills as possible. When a large number of medications must be taken, discontinue all unnecessary drugs and attempt to prescribe pills of different size, shape and color.

5. From time to time, ask the high-risk patient if he has any questions or concerns about the illness or its treatment if he does not volunteer matters of concern.

6. Do not discuss every possible side effect with all patients. Although a fully informed patient usually is in a better position to understand and cooperate with therapy, some patients become so preoccupied with rare side effects that they are afraid to take the medication. The physician therefore must decide with which patients he will discuss possible adverse effects in great detail (e.g., the patient with a need to be in control), and which ones should simply be told to report any new or unusual symptoms. When a side effect is discussed, the patient should be reassured that it will be treated promptly or the drug will be changed.

7. Ask the patient what he expects from treatment. Patients who do not feel treated without a particular medication, injection, or cultural remedy may not comply with a treatment in which they do not believe.

8. Maintain a high index of suspicion for noncompliance. Suspect this problem whenever a patient does not respond to treatment as expected, has not responded in the past, admits to having been noncompliant in the past, or has an illness that is likely to be associated with non-compliance because it is asymptomatic, chronic, or requires long-term therapy.

9. Ask the patient and his family if he is finding it difficult to follow the treatment plan. Little will be gained by hoping that the problem will resolve itself without open discussion or by waiting for the patient to bring up the topic.

10. Enlist the family's aid in securing compliance.
Demented patients or those with visual or hearing
losses who cannot keep track of their medications
almost always need someone else to monitor their
intake, and many patients who are afraid of treatment
can be reassured by family members.

11. Maintain a nonjudgmental attitude when noncompliance
is discovered. An angry, punitive approach is likely
to make the patient feel guilty and embarrassed,
causing him to conceal his nonadherence instead of
discussing it openly.

12. Be willing to compromise. When strong objections to one
aspect of the treatment plan are present, it may be
realistic not to insist that the patient adhere in return
for concessions on the patient's part. For example,
the patient with a recent M.I. who cannot tolerate
inactivity might be talked into staying in the hospital
in return for the physician's allowing him to be up
ad lib. Compromising with the patient makes him feel
more in control of the doctor-patient relationship and
helps him to assume more active responsibility for
himself.

13. Do not accede to demands that dangerously compromise
the physician's ability to be helpful. Some patients
refuse to engage in any therapeutic endeavor unless the
physician agrees either to do something that places the
patient or the physician in jeopardy (e.g., prescribe
large doses of narcotics) or not to do something that
would be necessary to preserve the patient's life or health
(e.g., not hospitalize the patient if he becomes suicidal).
Most of these demands have as their covert goal the
undoing of the physician's therapeutic usefulness, and
the primary clinician should obtain psychiatric consultation
before even considering agreeing to them. In the long
run, physician and patient may be better off never
entering into a potentially destructive doctor-patient
relationship, even if the alternative is no treatment at all.

REGRESSION

Consider a later development in Mrs. R.'s illness. She was able to stay in the hospital and gradually began to accept the possibility of having a serious illness. Further workup revealed acute leukemia, and chemotherapy was instituted. Then, the patient seems to undergo a personality change. She becomes irritable and complains constantly. Her ability to tolerate frustration and pain decreases dramatically, and she bursts into tears if she experiences nausea after receiving chemotherapy. She rings for the nurses incessantly, and never seems satisfied with the care she receives. Although she originally encouraged her husband to go home and look after the children, she now cannot stand to have him out of her sight. Additional history reveals that the patient was the third of seven children of a farming family. She helped to care for the younger children and worked on the farm in addition to going to school. She married at age nineteen, and one year later had her first child. Her husband describes her as a very independent, unselfish person, who hardly ever complains and who is always more interested in others' welfare than her own. He is surprised and frightened by her current behavior.

THE PHYSICIAN'S REACTION TO HIS PATIENT

At first glance, the patient's behavior may seem psychotic, and it is understandable that different psychiatric disorders, including schizophrenia and depression, are considered at this point. Some physicians feel that the patient is acting like an irascible child, and that what she really needs is a good spanking. This is not entirely inappropriate, since the patient is acting in a child-like manner: low frustration tolerance, complaining, crying when hurt, and low tolerance for separation are all normally seen in children who become ill. Physicians who view this behavior as normal may be denying the disturbance in order to avoid being upset by it.

COMMON UNSUCCESSFUL APPROACHES

Working with a patient who does not seem to be functioning on an adult level can be frustrating and confusing. Following are some common attempts to manage the regressed patient, with the patient's response and an explanation of the patient's behavior.

Physician's Approach	Patient's Response	Explanation
Tell the patient that she should be ashamed of herself for acting the way she does	The patient's behavior worsens	The patient's regression is a means of reducing the anxiety and embarrassment she feels about having to be cared for. Increasing her embarrassment increases her regression
Tell the patient to control herself and act like a grown-up	The patient attempts to "act normally" but is unable to do so	Since the patient's behavior is caused by a return to a child-like level of psychological functioning that is outside of her conscious control, her attempts to force herself to act differently are unsuccessful
Prescribe an antipsychotic drug	The patient becomes acutely agitated	Because the drug impairs the patient's ability to observe and control her own behavior, any remaining adult controls are diminished and she becomes even less capable of controlling her behavior

A SUCCESSFUL APPROACH

Every child goes through a long period of dependency. The normal child develops increasing independence as he matures, but is able to receive more caretaking at special times, even as an adult. For example, no one thinks it odd that a college student brings his laundry home on vacations or allows his mother to cook and otherwise care for him at these times, and the right of adults to be dependent when they are sick, injured or have experienced emotional trauma is codified in the sick role.

When (often because of illness, other hardship, or parental unwill- ingness) a child is not cared for normally, he may have to ignore his normal dependency needs and prematurely become independent. One means of achieving this goal is to deny his need to be cared for by deciding that he is much too busy taking care of other people to worry about himself. He may then become an excessively independent adult, who prides himself on his ability to take care of others, even at the expense of his own needs.

When such an individual becomes ill and needs care himself, the dependency needs that have been denied since childhood and therefore never integrated with the patient's adult personality break through with a child-like quality. Because the patient's behavior is so out of character for him, it confuses and embarrasses him, and he may even feel that he is losing his mind. Similar reactions may be observed in excessively dependent people whose already uncontrolled dependency is stimulated by being sick. In either case, regression usually is an acute reaction to the emotional stress of being ill and resolves with it.

An approach that takes these factors into account involves meeting the patient at his current level of functioning, while remembering that regression is a temporary reaction that usually resolves quickly:

1. Tell the patient that he is not losing his mind, but is experiencing a reaction to his illness that will resolve as he improves.

2. Set limits on the patient's behavior as one would a
   small child's. For example, if the patient refuses
   medication, tell him that he must take his medicine
   as prescribed. If he keeps ringing for the nurse,
   tell him firmly to stop.

3. As would a child, the patient can be expected to
   forget interventions regularly. Therefore, remind
   him frequently of the limits placed on his behavior.

4. Encourage unrestricted visiting by family members and
   close friends.

5. If the patient must be physically inactive (e.g., M.I.,
   burn, or post-operative patients), encourage some form
   of mental activity to lessen the patient's sense of
   passivity and the resultant regression. For example,
   reading, building a model, or playing a game such as
   cards or chess, involve more mental activity than watching
   T.V. or listening to the radio.

6. Do not delay medically indicated discharge because
   the patient is regressed and seems unable to tolerate
   leaving the hospital. Discharging the patient despite
   his protest usually reverses the regression.

7. Obtain psychiatric consultation for chronically ill
   patients who are regressed. Because these patients'
   illnesses do not remit, regression is likely to be more
   longstanding.

THE DYING PATIENT

The psychological management of the dying patient is a complex and
demanding task that challenges the physician's sensitivity and skill.
Consider, for example, the additional problem now posed by Mrs. R:
Although she does not look severely ill, it is clear that her long-term
prognosis is poor. She has not discussed her diagnosis or outlook for
the future.

The physician knows that, before she is discharged, her illness and its prognosis should be discussed. However, when he is confronted with the patient, her husband, and their two young children, all of whom seem cheerful at the prospect of the patient's going home, he is unsure how to proceed.

THE PHYSICIAN'S REACTION TO HIS PATIENT

Strong reactions to dying patients in the people caring for them are very common. If an attempt is made to ignore these feelings, they may be expressed in action instead of words. In the left-hand column below are some common reactions to dying patients, opposite comments on their significance.

Physician's Reaction	*Comments*
Feeling like a failure	Exposure in medical school to acutely ill patients and to patients the student does not follow over time leads many new physicians to assume that good medical care should result in a cure, and that if the patient does not recover or dies the physician must somehow be to blame. This feeling may be mixed with anger with the patient for not recovering and at oneself for not saving the patient
Feeling that little can be done to help the patient besides just offering psychological support	The sense of helplessness stemming from the physician's inability to <u>cure</u> the patient may make him feel that nothing can be done to <u>help</u> her. However, the proper psychological intervention can accomplish a great deal and provide a rewarding experience for both patient and physician

Physician's Reaction	Comments
Assuming that the patient should be left alone to deal with her problems	Avoiding the dying patient emotionally or physically is a way of avoiding the strong feelings of sadness, helplessness, hopelessness, and fear of death aroused by close contact with her
Sadness	Anyone who works closely with a dying patient and develops human feelings for her can expect to feel sad at the thought of losing her. These feelings may be especially intense if the doctor is reminded of other people he has lost or has become particularly attached to the patient

COMMON UNSUCCESSFUL APPROACHES

The left-hand column below lists commonly used approaches to the dying patient that are unlikely to be helpful. The middle column describes the patient's response, and the right-hand column provides an explanation for the patient's behavior.

Physician's Approach	Patient's Response	Explanation
Put the patient in a single room at the end of the hallway, so she will not upset the other patients or be upset by them	The patient becomes withdrawn and depressed	The patient already feels isolated from the world of the living. Separating her from nursing staff and other patients increases her sense of isolation. She also may conclude that, because she is ill, she does not deserve to be near other people

Physician's Approach	*Patient's Response*	*Explanation*
Attempt to avoid worrying the patient by not telling her the diagnosis	The patient becomes depressed, anxious and hopeless	Sooner or later, most terminal patients deduce that they have a terminal illness. Failure to discuss this diagnosis openly creates estrangement from the doctor, and makes the patient feel that he does not consider her competent to deal with reality or does not respect her enough to be honest. She also may feel that, if the doctor cannot deal with her illness openly, she will certainly be unable to handle it
Tell the patient that since she has a terminal illness, nothing more can be done for her	The patient becomes suicidal	Since the patient cannot expect to live a normal life span, the hope that she can accomplish something in what remains of her life is crucial if she is to separate her illness from other aspects of her life. Telling the patient that nothing more can be done for her implies that her life is already over and the patient may see no reason to continue living
Begin to discuss the patient's right to die a dignified death, and plan the circumstances under which life support will be terminated	The patient becomes preoccupied with death, and pays less attention to her family, her husband, and other everyday matters	While this is an appropriate topic at some point in the patient's course, a much more immediate problem is how the patient will live. Living with a terminal illness often involves grief at giving up loved ones, goals, and hopes for the future. This painful experience and other problems of living are sometimes avoided by focusing on death rather than life

Physician's Approach	Patient's Response	Explanation
Refer the patient immediately to a psychiatrist or clergyman to discuss the psychological or spiritual aspects of dying	An inpatient sees the consultant but tells him nothing. An outpatient agrees to referral but never makes an appointment	The patient feels that her illness creates a defect in her which inspires other people (including doctors) to avoid her. Sending her to a consultant before a trusting relationship is established with her own doctor may increase her feeling that her physician is unable or unwilling to help her with her emotions. She then agrees that emotions are not worth facing and, afraid of losing her primary doctor, avoids the consultant

A SUCCESSFUL APPROACH

The news that a patient has a terminal illness imposes several crucial psychological tasks during the remainder of the patient's life:

1. The patient must set his affairs in order to provide for those he will leave behind.

2. He must begin to say goodbye to the people who are close to him. The grief that the dying patient experiences over losing the living is as real as that experienced by the survivors who are losing him.

3. The realization that his life will not continue indefinitely forces him to reassess his goals and hopes for himself in a more immediate light. He may have to acknowledge that he cannot accomplish some of the tasks he thought he might get to eventually, and admit that he has not lived up to all of his expectations of himself. For example, the patient who has felt for years that when he had the time he would go back to school, must now face the fact that this dream will never be realized.

4. The patient also must decide whether he will attend
    to important matters which he has been putting off.
    For example, the man who has always meant to have
    a heart-to-heart talk with his son must now attempt
    to do so or forever lose the opportunity. Often,
    great progress is made in changing patterns of
    behavior when the patient has the knowledge that
    he will not get another chance to change.

5. He must review his accomplishments and failures and
    begin to come to a conclusion about how meaningful
    his life has been.

6. The patient must live with pain, disfigurement,
    limitation of activity, helplessness, and fear of
    abandonment, in a way that preserves his self-respect
    and sense of competence.

Facing these tasks can cause considerable psychological upheaval,
and it is not surprising that many people attempt to avoid them. As
the patient begins to adapt to his illness, he may demonstrate any or
all of the following reactions:

1. Denial is common throughout the patient's course. It
    provides the patient with a means of dealing with
    powerful feelings without being overwhelmed. Denial
    may be followed by a period of acknowledgement of the
    severity of the illness, which in turn may be followed
    by more denial, until the patient gradually comes to
    accept the illness and its consequences.

2. The patient feels anger at himself for being sick, at
    doctors and hospital staff for not curing him, and at
    family, friends and even strangers, for being healthy
    and having a normal life span. This often provokes
    anger in return from doctors, nursing staff, family
    and friends.

3. Depression occurs in reaction to loss of health, body
    parts, independence, control, self-esteem, and
    anticipated loss of life and loved ones.

4. Anxiety arises at the prospect of permanent separation
    from loved ones, and the prospect of being helpless to
    control pain and the course of the illness.

5. The patient may attempt to <u>bargain</u> for extra time in an attempt to regain some sense of control over his life, as though he had the power to ask for concessions.

6. A process of <u>dehumanization</u> may occur, which may be aggravated by his doctors' attending excessively to medical procedures without paying enough attention to him as a person.

7. The patient feels <u>detachment</u> from the world of the living and expresses the wish to be left alone to think. As he begins to come to terms with his illness and to say goodbye to loved ones, the sense of detachment increases. As opposed to depressive withdrawal, which is associated with anger, unhappiness and a sense of not having completed important tasks, detachment is accompanied by a sense of acceptance.

When the illness itself cannot be cured, a great deal still can be accomplished as the physician helps the patient to make the remainder of his life as physically comfortable and psychologically meaningful as possible. The following guidelines can help the clinician to achieve these goals:

1. Be truthful with the patient. Explain the diagnosis simply and explicitly. If he has questions, answer them directly.

2. If the patient does not seem to understand the diagnosis, even after it has been carefully explained, he may not be ready to accept the news that he has a fatal illness. In this case, do not attempt to force the realization upon him. When the patient feels ready, he will begin to ask questions about his diagnosis or treatment, or otherwise indicate that he wishes to discuss his illness and its meaning in greater depth.

3. Some patients continue to deny awareness of the seriousness of their illness until the day they die even though they cooperate with medical care and attend at least to some of the important tasks of dying. Usually, little is gained by confronting this denial.

4. Treat pain with adequate doses of narcotics,
    without fear of creating addiction. Cancer patients
    in particular may be able to tolerate extremely
    high doses of analgesics.

5. Accept the range of emotional reactions experienced
    by the patient and discuss them openly with him.
    The patient may attempt to hide these reactions
    (especially anger at the doctor) because he is afraid
    of alienating the physician. Encouraging him to
    talk about his feelings will relieve the pressure
    they cause, and sharing them will decrease the
    patient's sense of isolation.

6. Do not discourage hope about the future even if it
    seems unrealistic. Patients may talk about having a
    fatal illness, and in the next breath speak as though
    they had a normal lifespan. This represents a normal
    mixture of reality testing, denial, and hope.

7. It is equally important to avoid attempting to bolster
    false hope with empty encouragements such as, "a cure
    for your disease might be just around the corner."
    The patient will sense that these comments are designed
    to stop him from talking about dying and to reassure
    the physician.

8. Involve the patient's family in the process of
    diagnosis and treatment. If they seem reluctant to
    become involved, they may be afraid of the mourning
    process they will have to go through in giving him
    up. Open discussion of their concerns and respect
    for their concerns may make it easier for them to support
    the patient. If the family is still uninvolved,
    psychiatric intervention may be useful in delineating
    the reason.

9. If the patient is hospitalized, ask him if he would
    like a roommate and, if so, provide one. Prevent
    him from becoming isolated from the nursing staff by
    encouraging frequent visits and open discussion with
    them.

10. Treat depression vigorously, as in a patient with a normal lifespan. The temptation to accept suicidal thoughts as reflecting the "right to die with dignity" (an entirely separate issue) should be avoided.

11. Communicate the attitude that even though the dying patient cannot be cured, a great deal can be accomplished in what remains of his life to add meaning and richness to it. If the doctor views terminal illness as providing opportunities for personal growth, his courage and enthusiasm will be communicated to the patient.

12. Remember that most people die as they live and that dying brings out the best in some individuals and the worst in others. Do not demand more of the patient than he is capable of achieving on the grounds that all longstanding problems should be worked through before one dies.

13. Working with the emotional worlds of dying patients invariably evokes strong feelings in the physician which can be tolerated more easily with the support of colleagues, family and friends. To avoid "burnout," the physician also may wish to limit himself to working intensively with the psychological reactions of only one or two dying patients at a time, and to allow himself to grieve after he has lost a patient with whom he has worked closely.

GRIEF

Acute grief is a normal syndrome which appears after a significant loss, e.g., of a loved one, body part, health, function, income, status, or even of a place to which one has become attached. Grief represents the process by which the emotional investment to the lost person, thing, etc., is gradually withdrawn, so that new attachments can be formed. Stronger attachments naturally evoke more intense grief when they are broken. Grief roughly follows three stages, which will be described with respect to loss of a person:

1. There is a period of <u>disbelief</u> characterized by denial
   of the emotional impact of the loss, and sometimes
   of the loss itself. This period serves a protective
   function, allowing the patient to prepare himself for
   the impact of the loss. It lasts a few minutes to
   a few days, and reappears from time to time throughout
   the mourning process.

2. <u>Working through</u> feelings of loss for the person who
   has died begins minutes to days after the death, as
   the patient begins the process of saying goodbye.
   It peaks in 4-6 weeks, is intense for about 3 months,
   and gradually subsides over 6-12 months, but may
   normally last a number of years. Prominent symptoms
   during this period include the following:

   - <u>Painful preoccupation with the deceased</u> appears,
     abates, and then reappears in response to
     thinking or talking about him, receiving
     sympathy, or anything that reminds the patient
     of the deceased. It is accompanied by sadness
     and crying

   - <u>Anxiety and restlessness</u>, with physiologic signs
     of arousal (shortness of breath, tachycardia,
     hyperventilation, etc.), often is accompanied
     by an urge to search for the lost person and
     by the conviction that he will appear at any
     moment

   - <u>Generalized somatic distress</u>, especially choking
     sensations, headaches, anorexia, insomnia, GI
     complaints, and weakness are expressions of a
     sense of physical as well as mental disorganization

   - <u>Anger</u> may be directed at family and friends
     (for still being alive), the doctor (for not
     curing the patient), the deceased (for dying),
     and even at God for allowing the death to occur

   - <u>Guilt</u> usually is restricted to thoughts about
     ways in which the patient should have behaved
     differently toward the deceased, feelings that
     the patient could have saved him, or a conviction
     that the patient should have died instead. It is
     not as pervasive as the guilt of depression and is
     not accompanied by loss of self-esteem

- <u>Identification phenomena</u> represent an
  unconscious mimicking of the deceased by
  developing similar physical symptoms (e.g.,
  headaches appearing in the widow of a man
  who died of a CVA), or taking on his behavior
  patterns. These symptoms represent a means
  of keeping part of the lost person inside
  the patient

- <u>Disorganization</u> of usual patterns of behavior
  makes it difficult for the patient to function
  normally at work or recreational activities

- Transient auditory or visual <u>hallucinations</u>
  of the deceased are normal expressions of
  intense grief, but may be very frightening
  to the patient

3. Resolution of grieving and <u>resumption of normal</u>
   <u>functioning</u> begins after about six to twelve months,
   as symptoms gradually abate. Sadness, painful
   memories, and longing for the deceased recur
   periodically, especially on anniversaries and other
   significant dates such as holidays or birthdays.

Grief now becomes an issue for Mrs. R's family. She achieved a
remission after chemotherapy was instituted, and was able to carry
on a relatively normal life for some time. Symptoms of regression were
not prominent during subsequent hospitalizations, and the patient
exhibited great courage in the face of considerable suffering. She was
a source of support for her family, and was liked by everyone who took
care of her. During her last hospitalization, she gradually sank into
a coma and died. At the request of the patient and her husband, heroic
resuscitation measures were not attempted.

A few days later, Mr. R stops by. The ensuing conversation is
remarkably different from the physician's previous interactions with
him:

Pt: I wanted to talk about the decision not to resuscitate
     my wife...I've been wondering if we really did the
     right thing.

Dr: Well, we all discussed it many times before she died.

Pt: Yes, but I really wonder...don't you think you
could have kept her alive a while longer, at least
until a new treatment came along?

Dr: I wish there were a cure, but I don't think she
could have been saved.

Pt: How can you be so sure? Maybe I should have consulted
with another physician. I don't know if I did the
right thing and I'm not sure you really helped us.
What about the new treatment for leukemia I read about
yesterday? I have some real questions about whether
this case was handled right.

THE PHYSICIAN'S REACTION TO HIS PATIENT

When the physician has worked hard to help a patient who dies, it
may be especially upsetting when a family member's request for assistance with his own feelings takes the form of an attack on the doctor.
Common reactions to such situations are listed below, opposite comments
on their significance.

Physician's Reaction	*Comments*
Anger at the survivor	This is an understandable reaction toward someone who attacks a physician who tried his hardest to prolong the patient's life. If the clinician is beginning to mourn the loss of the patient himself, he also may resent the survivor's insistence that the doctor attend to his distress while avoiding his own sadness by becoming angry

Physician's Reaction	*Comments*
Wish to defend oneself against criticisms of the quality of medical care	Even if the physician knows that he has done a good job, his sense of guilt at not having cured the patient may lead him to feel that the family member's accusations may be correct and to attempt to defend himself from their (and his own) criticisms
Feeling helpless and overwhelmed	Dealing with strong emotions of anger or the sadness behind it may seem like an overwhelming task to the physician who has reactions of his own to the patient's death, especially if he feels that the chances of dealing constructively with feelings related to the patient's illness are as remote as was the hope of curing her
Sadness	The doctor feels an empathic response to the survivor's underlying grief, perhaps mixed with his own grief at losing a patient to whom he had come to feel attached

COMMON UNSUCCESSFUL APPROACHES

The physician may attempt to reduce the grieving patient's psychological pain by reassuring him and telling him that he should not feel bad. However, interrupting active mourning prolongs the grief process, makes the bereaved feel that his feelings are intolerable, and may convert grief to depression. If the physician feels that he does not deserve the survivor's anger, or that the survivor is not his patient, he may avoid further contact with him. Angry, nonproductive encounters are likely to continue if the physician responds to the patient's attack with anger of his own.

A SUCCESSFUL APPROACH

Grief is treated by helping the survivor to begin the process of mourning. In Mr. R's case, anger on the surface is related to the mourning process in several ways:

1. He may feel angry at his wife for leaving him. Since it was not the wife's fault for dying, the survivor then feels that his anger is unjustified and anger may then be displaced (moved) onto the doctor, against whom it feels easier to justify.

2. His anger at the doctor may represent an attempt to disguise from himself his own guilt at not having done more for his wife while she was alive. He also may have wished at some point that her life would end so that her suffering, as well as his own misery at waiting for her to die, would stop. His guilt at these feelings then is projected onto the physician so that he can avoid recognizing it in itself.

3. As long as the survivor feels angry, he avoids the painful sadness of grieving for his wife.

The doctor may help the survivor to begin the grieving process by gently pointing out the meaning of his anger, by encouraging him to pay attention to his sadness, and by reassuring him that he will feel better if he faces his grief:

Dr: You must miss your wife terribly.

Pt: Of course I do--thanks to you.

Dr: It makes you very angry not to have her with you anymore.

Pt: Why couldn't she have lived just a little longer?

Dr: I wish she were alive, too. I think it's very sad that she's dead.

Pt: I can't let myself feel that...I've got to carry
     on...to take care of the kids...

Dr: It's frightening to think about your sadness; but
     facing your feelings about your wife won't be over-
     whelming. Your children can share in your grief,
     and I can help you all with it. As hard as it may
     seem to you now, you can deal with your sadness
     and feel better.

Pt: I've felt so sad--(starts to cry)

At this point the doctor should allow the patient some time to
begin expressing his sadness, conveying in action the physician's understanding and willingness to work with the patient's grief.

After the survivor has acknowledged his grief, the following
guidelines apply:

1. Meet with the patient regularly for 20 minutes or so
    once or twice a week, telling him in advance how long
    sessions will last and how frequently they will occur.

2. Explain that grief is a necessary process that
    necessarily involves emotional pain; however, if the
    survivor continues to express his emotions he will
    gradually feel better.

3. Ask the survivor to tell the doctor about the deceased
    and their life together.

4. Some symptoms of normal grief may be especially disturbing,
    including difficulty carrying out everyday tasks and
    relationships, anger, guilt, identification symptoms,
    and hallucinations. If the survivor is worried by these
    symptoms, reassure him that they are part of the grief
    process and do not necessarily indicate a psychosis.

5. If the patient has a great deal of difficulty sleeping,
    an H.S. sleeping medication such as flurazepam (Dalmane)
    or temazepam (Restoril) may be prescribed.

6. Day-time sedation of any kind should be avoided, as it serves to suppress symptoms of grief and prolong the mourning process. Unless clear symptoms of depression (e.g., pervasive sense of guilt, lowered self-esteem, vegetative signs, etc.) are present, antidepressants also should be avoided.

7. Children should be provided with the chance to share in the family's grief. Explaining the death simply and honestly, and encouraging the child to express his feelings usually is indicated, and the rest of the family should feel free to express their emotions in front of the children. Excluding children from the mourning process robs them of the opportunity to work through their feelings and isolates them from the rest of the family at the time they need them the most. Euphemisms that should be avoided in discussing the death of a parent or sibling include:

- "Mommy's gone on a trip." The child will keep expecting her to come back.

- "Mommy is watching over us." This serves to confuse and frighten the child, who thinks that his mother watches every bad thing that he does.

- "Mommy is living in heaven." The child will not understand why she does not want to live with him. Also, his grieving will be cut short as he will think that she is still alive.

COMPLICATIONS OF GRIEF

If the survivor expresses his feelings about the person who has died and mentally reviews their relationship, the symptoms of grief abate over six months to a year as he gradually gives up the deceased. He will then be able to engage in new, rewarding relationships. When this process does not occur normally, pathological forms of grief may occur. These include the following:

1. Inhibited grief occurs when the patient does not
   allow himself to experience any grief, and
   consciously is unaware of any sadness. However,
   somatic complaints, difficulty carrying on the
   normal interactions in which he previously engaged,
   insomnia and even identification symptoms may be
   experienced for years.

2. Delayed grief occurs months to years after a death
   when some event, e.g., the anniversary of the death,
   precipitates active grieving that previously had
   been suppressed.

3. Chronic anger may occur in place of grief, often
   directed at doctors or other family members. The
   survivor may even threaten to sue for malpractice,
   but rarely carries out such threats if the physician
   does not become angry in return.

4. Chronic grief ("reactive" depression) occurs when
   markedly mixed (ambivalent) feelings in the relationship
   with the deceased make giving him up complicated. This
   occurs, for example, if the survivor feels extremely
   angry at the person who has died (e.g., in a suicide),
   if the relationship was characterized by intense anger
   as well as love, or if the survivor wished that the
   patient would die. When symptoms of pervasive guilt,
   lowered self-esteem, and vegetative signs appear, or
   when acute grief does not begin to resolve within a
   few months, depression has supervened.

5. Precipitation of a psychiatric disorder, e.g., schizophrenia,
   may occur in patients predisposed to develop such disorders.

6. Alcoholism and/or drug abuse may represent a chronic
   attempt to suppress grief.

7. Precipitous remarriage may occur in an attempt to
   suppress all feelings about a deceased spouse by replacing
   her with someone else.

8. Some authors feel that medical and psychosomatic illnesses
   may be precipitated by a loss in vulnerable individuals.
   For example, increased mortality from cardiovascular
   disease occurs in older widowers in the 6 months following
   a loss.

While it is not possible to predict with certainty those people who will have complicated grief reactions, factors that place the survivor at increased risk include:

1. Delay of more than 2 weeks in onset of active grieving

2. Ambivalent relationship with the deceased

3. Death occurred under unusual or complicated circumstances (e.g., suicide)

4. No opportunity to prepare for the loss (e.g., after a sudden, unexpected death)

5. Lack of emotional supports other than the deceased in the survivor's life

6. Inability to tolerate or express emotions

7. History of past unresolved losses

8. History of loss of a significant person in childhood

9. Past history of depression

10. Past history or family history of other serious psychiatric disorder (e.g., schizophrenia, mania)

USE OF THE PSYCHIATRIST

An increasing number of centers provide ongoing psychiatric consultation to medical and surgical services. These psychiatric liaison services provide consultees with the opportunity to discuss not only diagnostic problems and reactions of patients to their illnesses, but also issues that may affect physicians' and nurses' ability to deliver effective care. These services may be utilized in the following ways:

The physician should consult with a psychiatrist if:

1. The patient has a past history of a stormy emotional course during an illness

2. Forces impinging on the physician or nurses (e.g., personal problems similar to those of the patient, excess administrative stress) may affect the patient's management

3. The patient denies that he is sick at all

4. The physician or nurses wish help devising a treatment plan

5. A treatment plan is unsuccessful

6. A severe psychiatric disorder may be present

7. The patient requests some dangerous compromise as a prerequisite to treatment

8. The patient is at risk of complicated grief

9. The family's reaction to the patient's illness is complicated

10. The physician finds it difficult to control his reaction to the patient

The physician should refer the patient to a psychiatrist if:

1. The patient develops a psychotic reaction to his illness

2. The patient is difficult to manage on an open medical floor (e.g., agitated or suicidal patients)

3. The patient engages in self-destructive, noncompliant behavior

4. The patient is poorly motivated to alter noncompliant behavior

5. The physician does not wish to take primary responsibility for managing the emotional component of the patient's illness

REFERENCES

Becker E: The Denial of Death. New York, Free Press, 1973

Boucharlat J: Hospitalization and Regression. Ann Med Psychol (Paris) 1974; 2:582

Foster JR, et al: To die young, to die old: management of terminal illness at age 20 and age 85. J Geriat Psychiatry 1975; 8:111

Kahana RJ, Bibring GL: Personality Types in Medical Management. In: Zinberg NE: Psychiatry and Medical Practice in a General Hospital. New York, International Universities Press, 1964 pp 108-123

Krupp NE: Adaptation to chronic illness. Postgrad Med 1976; 60:122

Kubler-Ross E: On Death and Dying. New York, MacMillan, 1969

Mecham D: Illness behavior, social adaptation and the management of illness. J Nerv Ment Dis 1977; 165:79

Miller WB: A Psychophysiological Study of Denial Following Acute M.I. J Psychosom Res 1975; 19:43

Parkes CM: Bereavement. New York, International Universities Press, 1972

White RB: The Syndrome of Ordinary Grief. Am Fam Physician 1973; 8:97

Chapter Seven

FAMILY PROBLEMS

by Ruth Fuller, M.D.

An illness never involves only one person; it evolves within the context of the patient's social world, usually his family. Other people can have a profound effect, not only on the patient's adaptation to his disease, but also on how quickly or even whether he recovers. At the same time, an individual's illness can have an integrating or destabilizing effect on other family members. Although these multiple interactions initially may seem complex, the family can be of vital assistance in history taking and treatment planning, and their help may be essential in obtaining the patient's compliance. However, family concerns may not be apparent to the physician because the family hides them out of embarrassment or a fear of being considered abnormal. Unless these issues are addressed, family anxiety remains unnecessarily high and the family may be an impediment, rather than an ally, in the patient's medical care. Families commonly experience the following overt or covert concerns:

1. Guilt. Family members may feel that they have contributed to the patient's illness, particularly if they were angry at the patient before he got sick.

2. Anger. Resentment at the patient for becoming ill is a common concern, especially if the illness causes drastic changes in the family's circumstances. It often is not expressed directly because family members do not think it right to become angry with someone who cannot help being ill.

3. Anxiety and feelings of helplessness. The family may deal with their own fears about the patient's illness in a manner analagous to the ways in which individuals handle anxiety (see pp 65-70).

4. Pleasure. A particularly guilt-provoking reaction is a sense of gratification at the patient's suffering as other family members feel they have suffered.

5. Relief. Severely dysfunctional families may seek hospitalization for one member in order to relieve unbearable tensions and remove attention from problems in other family members.

6. Disruption of established roles. Family members may
    have depended on the patient to be an independent
    caretaker and may be unprepared to take care of him,
    as well as to assume more independence themselves.

CLUES TO THE DIAGNOSIS OF FAMILY PROBLEMS

Families respond to the stress of illness in characteristic ways.
Some become agitated, others withdrawn and isolated, and some become
disorganized, anxious or depressed. Following are indicators of family
difficulty that are cause for further investigation:

1. The physician is bombarded by telephone calls and
    messages from worried family members

2. The family does not seem to understand the doctor's
    explanations and treatment plan

3. The family appears upset, angry, demanding or overly
    critical about the patient's medical care

4. Family members demonstrate an inappropriate lack
    of concern

5. No one visits the hospitalized patient

6. History taking reveals that no one seems to know
    much about other family members' lives

7. Family members are self-critical about the patient's
    illness, e.g., "If only I had not argued with my
    husband he would not have fallen ill"

8. Appointments are missed, prescriptions are not
    filled or medications are given incorrectly

9. A child develops trouble with the law, fights,
    school phobia, truancy, multiple accidents, drug
    or alcohol abuse, or other obvious signs of distress

10. Family arguments increase or decrease

11.   Family members appear not to want the patient to be
      seen alone by the doctor

12.   Healthy family members develop unexplained somatic
      complaints

13.   Any family member seems depressed or anxious

ENCOUNTER WITH A TYPICAL FAMILY

Mr. F. is a 53-year-old man who was admitted to the neurology
service on an emergency basis. Earlier that evening, following an
argument with his wife, he suddenly collapsed at home.

Mr. and Mrs. F. are native to the area, always having lived
within 20 miles of their respective parents. Mr. F., a very successful
engineer, has always been in good physical health and has never been
hospitalized before. Mrs. F. is a fulltime wife and mother. The
children attend local high schools and colleges, and are excellent
students.

While Mr. F. is being evaluated, Mrs. F. and her three
children bombard the housestaff and nurses with questions concerning
Mr. F.'s condition and the cause of his sudden collapse. For the
resident physician attempting to obtain a history and reassure the
family, the task approaches the impossible:

Dr: We think that your husband has had a cerebrovascular
      accident. A blood vessel in the brain was weak and
      then ruptured...

Mrs. F: (interrupting) Is he all right? When can I take
      him home?

Dr: We are in the process...

Mrs. F: But is he all right? Will he be all right? Was
      it something he ate?

Dr: At this point...

Oldest son: Doctor, my mother asked if my father will
      be all right.

Dr: We're doing our best. Let me...

Mrs. F: (crying) What's going to happen to us? Has a
real doctor seen him?

Dr: Well...

Mrs. F: Could it be a virus? He wasn't feeling very
well last week.

Dr: I don't.think so. But we're doing everything we can.

Mrs. F: How can you be doing everything if you're not sure
what's wrong?

THE PHYSICIAN'S REACTIONS TO THE FAMILY

Because the doctor belongs to a family himself, he can be expected
to have developed a number of ideas about how families work and how
they should be approached that may not apply to his patients. The
tendency to apply idiosyncratic methods when dealing with families is
intensified by the lack of adequate training in dealing with families
provided in medical school and the greater sense of dealing with only
one other person. Common reactions to the prospect of treating a
family are listed in the left-hand column below, while their significance
is discussed on the right.

Physician's Reaction	*Comment*
Conviction that working with families is unimportant or is more trouble than it is worth	The doctor understandably feels overwhelmed at the thought of having to deal with so many people who are upset at once and attempts to avoid the task by minimizing its importance
Feeling that the family is too angry to work constructively with the physician	Families, like individuals, may conceal anxiety under a facade of anger. Like most anxious individuals, they usually respond to a calm, confident approach and to empathy with their underlying fears

Physician's Reaction	*Comment*
Philosophy that dealing with families is the job of nurses and social workers	Particularly if the physician fears the family's criticism or feels unable to help them, he may wish to avoid working with them by defining this task as someone else's job

COMMON UNSUCCESSFUL APPROACHES

An interaction between two people is complex enough; the prospect of dealing with three, four or more people can seem staggering if the physician does not have at his disposal at least the same amount of confidence he feels with the individual patient. Following are some commonly applied unsuccessful attempts to work with families, along with the patient's or family's response and an explanation of the reasons why these responses occur:

Physician's Approach	*Patient/Family Response*	*Explanation*
Explain the nature of the illness and its expected course while attempting to ignore the family's agitation	No one listens to what the doctor has to say about the technical aspects of the case. The wife becomes increasingly frightened and demands the answer to one question: will her husband be all right? The son becomes angry and protective of his mother	Illness in any individual evokes fears in other family members, the most prominent of which often are concerns that the patient will die and that the family will be unable to function without him. When their concerns are not addressed directly, the family becomes convinced that the doctor is afraid to tell them that their worst fears will come true
Tell the family not to worry	The family becomes even more demanding and critical	Reassurance that is offered too rapidly without first uncovering the patient's specific concerns make the family feel that the physician cannot help them and their sense of being overwhelmed and frightened increases

Physician's Approach	*Patient/Family Response*	*Explanation*
Discount the wife's unlikely explanations of her husband's illness such as "it was something he ate" or "a virus"	The wife makes a suicide attempt	Family members are likely to feel guilty about the patient's illness, especially when unresolved emotional issues were present before the patient became ill. If Mrs. F. feels that she was responsible for her husband's illness because it occurred during a fight, she may attempt to reassure herself that she did not cause it by blaming it on other factors. Undercutting her attempt to avoid her sense of guilt without helping her to find a better way to deal with it may result in depression
Give information to one family member, telling him to "pass it on" to the others	The family becomes convinced that the patient is terminally ill	When a family's equilibrium is disrupted, individuals cannot be relied upon to avoid distorting information in the light of their own fears
Do not meet with the entire family. Instead, refer each person who seems to have a problem to a different psychiatrist or mental health professional	The family's criticism of the physician and each other increases	In a close-knit family, the thought of separation due to illness or the threat of death is especially frightening. Separate referral reinforces each family member's feeling of isolation, and they blame each other instead of providing mutual support. They also blame the physician for not helping them to approach their problems more constructively

A SUCCESSFUL APPROACH

Since the entire family, and not just the identified patient, must adapt to the patient's illness, the physician's task is to open lines of communication in a sympathetic, non-threatening manner and to help uncover covert family concerns. Initial resistances to discussing problems openly usually can be dealt with directly:

Dr: Could we get together and discuss your husband's illness?

Wife: Oh, I'm so busy, I don't know when I could.

Dr: You must have a lot more responsibility at home
      since your husband has been ill.

Wife: I really don't know how to handle it at all; there are
      so many things to do.

Dr: Maybe you feel you haven't been handling this whole
      situation well?

Wife: I've been tense constantly. I can't sleep, I'm angry,
      I yell at the children...anyway, you look very busy and
      I shouldn't bother you with my problems.

Dr: You know, the family's problem is the patient's problem,
      and that makes it my concern, too.

Wife: I've just felt so guilty about the way I've been
      behaving and about my not being able to control the kids.

Dr: I think the whole family has been upset by your husband's
      illness. You must have a number of questions about
      what's going on.

Wife: If we hadn't argued, none of this would have happened.
      It's all my fault.

Dr: It's understandable that you would worry that you caused
      your husband's stroke; but it was caused by an anatomical
      defect and not by your argument. But you and your family
      must have many other questions about your husband's
      illness that are bothering all of you. Why don't we
      all get together this evening to discuss these questions
      and the way you all have been feeling?

The physician has recognized that the entire family has a problem that is understandable and manageable and has made it clear that he

will help each member to express his concerns openly. When the family
meets he can restate the importance of their solving their problems as
a unit and help them to begin to express their fears, their anger at
the patient for being sick, their guilt for feeling angry at him, their
guilt about his illness, and their sense of isolation from each other.
When any family member expresses concerns openly, everyone feels less
isolated and group problem solving can begin.

The following guidelines are useful when working with families
around an illness that requires hospitalization:

1. Begin to develop a relationship with the family as early
   in the illness as possible. A brief introduction when
   the patient is admitted and a promise to meet with them
   as soon as the workup is completed is advisable in
   most cases.

2. At the initial meeting with the patient and his family,
   the physician has the opportunity to see who does most
   of the speaking for the family, the mood of each person,
   how they relate to each other, who appears to be an
   accurate listener or reporter, etc. Identifying
   responsible and cooperative family members is critical
   in obtaining an accurate history and planning treatment,
   as is finding those who are likely to subvert therapeutic efforts (e.g., by encouraging noncompliance).

3. Find out from the family who is working (when, where and
   with what flexibility); who is at home (when and with
   what responsibilities); and who is viewed by the patient
   as both desirable and available for help with daily
   care. Some families find it very difficult to make
   decisions concerning such matters as who will take care
   of the patient or offer support, without a good deal of
   guidance. Other families are quite organized in making
   these decisions, while in a few situations it may be
   difficult to determine who is able to be a caretaker
   and who needs to remain in a dependent role. A major
   task therefore is to clarify family roles and responsibilities.

4. With the patient present, explain to the family in
   detail the medical findings as well as the treatment
   plan in order to keep distortions to a minimum.

5. Convey to the family the physician's expectation that
   they will participate in the patient's care. If they
   express a wish to avoid meeting as a family, insist

firmly that they do so at least once, and then discuss the reasons why they are reluctant to participate.

6. Involve as many family members as possible, but always deal with those individuals who have assumed a leadership role during the patient's, illness. Even a child or distant relative may assume such a role if a healthy parent is unable to take parental responsibility.

7. Emphasize the importance of the family's sharing with each other any concerns about the illness. Encourage them to discuss with the physician any communication problems they experience.

8. See the family regularly - once a week for 10-15 minutes is enough when the acute phase of the illness has subsided. If the family is not having problems, they will be reassured by the doctor's continued presence. If problems develop, the doctor will be able to identify them quickly and begin more frequent meetings.

9. Instruct the ward staff to observe family interactions during visiting hours and note major changes.

10. During family meetings, encourage those individuals who remain silent to state their concerns openly, and limit those family members who monopolize the discussion. Even small children may be surprisingly eloquent when drawn out.

11. Prior to discharge, discuss the family's questions about what to expect when the patient comes home. It often is helpful to have the family contact the doctor shortly after discharge to let him know how they are doing. Consider followup family meetings on an outpatient basis to make sure that family adjustment is adequate.

OUTPATIENT TREATMENT

Families frequently consult the physician for help in negotiating crises that regularly arise in their development as a unit. Important nodal points in the life of a family include:

1. Marriage and the establishment of a new family unit

2. Birth of children, the development of parental roles and the reconciliation of these with professional goals

3. The beginning of the children's schooling

4. Emancipation of the children

5. Aging and chronic illness

6. Retirement

7. Death of friends and spouse

Crises with which families are likely to ask primary physicians for assistance often are associated with one of these nodal points. At these times, the following general guidelines apply:

1. Attempt to see the entire family together; but see anyone who is willing to appear.

2. Remain alert for the tendency of individuals to deal with guilt about problems having arisen by blaming each other for their difficulties.

3. Avoid identifying only one family member as the one with the problem. If the family identifies one member (the identified patient) as the only one experiencing difficulty, point out that this represents an attempt to avoid recognition of each person's responsibility for family difficulties and to shift attention away from painful emotions and conflicts in other family members.

4. Help the family to clarify its problems. Once the difficulty is diagnosed and unproductive anger and blaming each other is brought under control, the family often can do the rest.

5. Avoid taking sides or giving advice. Instead, assist
    the family in developing its own solutions.

6. Encourage all family members to participate in the
    discussion. If one person is silent, ask him why he
    does not talk.

7. If one family member dominates the discussion, ask the
    entire family why only one person is talking.

8. Interrupt destructive interactions and then ask all
    family members about their thoughts regarding the inter-
    action. For example, if a husband tells his wife to
    shut up and then begins to shout at her, stop him and
    ask him why he acts that way while asking the wife why
    she permits or encourages such behavior.

9. Ask about parents' or spouses' families of origin in
    an attempt to learn how destructive patterns were learned.

Examples of problems arising at specific developmental stages are:

1. _Marriage_. Families of origin may try to interfere with the
young couple's independence, resulting in frequent invitations to
participate in family activities without the spouse or in the parents
dropping in for unannounced visits. If the couple is reluctant to
strike out on their own, they may depend excessively on one or both sets
of parents for emotional or financial support. The couple may complain
directly about their difficulty establishing their own independence or
marital discord may signal this problem.

With increasing cultural acceptance, and even encouragement, of
cohabitation without marriage, couples who are afraid of committing themselves to each other may live together for long periods of time, only
to develop an acute disturbance in the relationship when marriage is
contemplated (often at a time when the couple is thinking about having
children). Anxiety, arguments and other problems when commitments are
formalized may be related to fear of depending on another person, reluctance to surrender autonomy, or a conviction that a person to whom one
becomes too close will leave or otherwise prove untrustworthy. Most
problems arising when a relationship begins in earnest respond to open
discussion of the couple's fears with a physician moderating the discussion and helping each partner to express his or her concerns in
words instead of action.

2. _Birth of the children_. Problems arising at this stage are
related to fears of becoming a parent, difficulty accepting parental
roles, and perceived conflicts between parenthood and a career,

especially in women. Ignorance about how to take care of a child,
unpleasant experiences with either partner's own parents, inability
to trust the other person and uncertainty about one's ability to
continue a career if time is taken away from the job to have a baby
predispose to difficulties when children are born. Common manifestations of difficulties assuming parenthood include:

- Arguments or uncertainty about how to manage the child

- Excessive concern about the child's health

- Repeated calls to the physician

- Jealousy by one parent of the time the other spends
  with the child

- Increasing amounts of time spent by one parent away
  from the home

- Beginning an extramarital affair

Management of these difficulties begins with a review with the
parents of normal childhood development, common childhood illnesses
and their symptoms, and normal feeding and sleeping patterns. It may
help to have the parents buy a parenting manual (e.g., "Dr. Spock")
that answers common questions asked by parents. In addition, if the
parents feel free to call the doctor at any time with whatever questions they have, their anxiety is likely to decrease. If reassurance,
support and correction of ignorance do not decrease the parents'
complaints, the physician should meet regularly with them to discuss
their concerns about assuming parental roles. If parents are ashamed
of having mixed feelings about parenthood they may not discuss them
with each other. They usually are relieved to find that their
partner understands and even has similar concerns, and that conflicts
about parenthood do not make one a bad parent. The physician should
evaluate child abuse potential when appropriate (see pp. 272-277).

3. <u>Growth of the children</u>. Problems arising at this stage often
result from parents' difficulties allowing their children increasing
autonomy and from childrens' ambivalence about accepting increasing
responsibilities for themselves. Common manifestations of this problem
include:

- Parents' bringing the child to the doctor to be talked out
  of a bad habit or a sport they consider dangerous

- Increasing arguments

- Rebelliousness in a teenager

- Inappropriate restrictions set forth by parents

Managing such problems requires that the doctor avoid siding with parent or child. If the parents insist that the doctor "straighten out" the child, the doctor can point out that they seem to be asking him to take over their role as parents. Next, the physician should encourage parents and child to discuss their differences of opinion openly, pointing out that parents often want their children to be independent but are reluctant to let go of them while children, no matter how much they wish to be independent, often are afraid of their new-found freedom.

4. The problem of aging and chronic illness often result in the need to discuss nursing home placement. Patients and their families have strikingly common fears about nursing homes, including:

- Nursing homes are places to die

- Families place relatives in nursing homes because the patient is no longer wanted by the family

- Nursing homes do not provide adequate care

- Once the patient is in a nursing home the family can no longer be involved in his care

The physician can be of great help in encouraging the family to broach a topic they consider unspeakable and in clarifying these incorrect assumptions. Nursing homes can provide nursing care in a less intense setting than the hospital but more than that which a family can provide. If the family does not have the expertise or manpower to provide extensive nursing care, making reasonable nursing home arrangements reflects how much they do care about the patient. If the placement is to be permanent, the doctor can help the family deal with the mixture of anguish, guilt and relief that frequently accompanies such decisions, while helping them to continue their involvement with the patient.

5. Retirement. Problems often develop after the children have left home, when either or both spouses retire, and when friends begin to die. Issues common to all these situations include grief for lost friends and for parent-child relationships that have changed in fundamental ways, fear of no longer being productive, and the parents'

need to relate to each other directly rather than through children,
friends and work. Often, hypochondriacal complaints and depression
signal the couple's wish for help in mastering these issues. The
physician can help the older couple by conveying a sense that aging
presents an opportunity for further growth, encouraging mourning of the
roles and relationships of a younger age, and asking about new
activities in which the couple might share. Couples whose relationship
requires a certain amount of distance may need to be helped to find
ways not to spend too much time with each other when leisure time
increases.

SPECIAL FAMILY PROBLEMS

Some family "secrets" exist that rarely are spoken about openly
but which nevertheless may be the real reason why the family seeks help
from the physician. These difficulties are particularly likely to be
missed when the doctor's reaction is overly moralistic, resulting in
the family's being even more anxious to conceal their problem. Some
common family secrets include:

1. Family collusion in maintaining silence even with
    each other, about incest, child abuse and family
    violence is characteristic. Once these problems are
    uncovered, reporting to the authorities
    is mandatory in many states if minors are involved.

2. Alcoholism usually is a well-kept family secret. Less
    than 5% of all problem drinkers resemble the stereotyped
    "alcoholic", while 95% have no obvious stigmata of the
    disease. However, undiagnosed alcoholism can complicate
    caring for any patient even if alcohol abuse is not
    directly related to the patient's presenting problem

3. Questions of paternity (or maternity) may be an unspoken
    but powerful dynamic. In the case of a different last
    name, the issue may be obvious. However, people
    frequently are ashamed about their origins and keep
    these concerns quiet. Nevertheless, a parent may
    harbor deep (and sometimes dangerous) resentment if
    he is convinced that a child is not his.

4. An adoption that the parents do not wish to acknowledge
    also can create family tensions and may be the cause of
    insecurity in children or parents, especially if one

spouse is unable to have children. The child's
questioning about such matters as the lack of baby
pictures or the story of the mother's pregnancy may
be blatantly ignored by the parents.

5. Teenage pregnancy has been increasing steadily. The
    physician should be alert to legal problems, drug abuse,
    truancy, depression or other difficulties that may arise
    because an adolescent is pregnant. The physician should
    understand his own attitude toward abortion, contra-
    ception, etc., and try not to impose his own beliefs on
    his patients. Wherever possible the goal should be to
    help parents and teenager solve this problem together.

6. Threatened divorce creates problems for everyone. The
    physician should avoid taking sides and help protect
    the children from becoming pawns in parental battles.
    He should avoid becoming a "messenger" between two
    arguing spouses, instead providing an arena in which
    opposing points of view can be discussed openly.

7. Illegal immigrant status is a growing issue which for
    obvious reasons is associated with the fear of discovery.
    Consequently, family members may be late in seeking
    medical care or provide vague or incomplete histories.
    Illegal aliens may be "captives" in low paying
    jobs and therefore live in poverty conditions that
    increase susceptibility to malnutrition and disease.

USE OF THE PSYCHIATRIST

The physician should consult with the psychiatrist if:

1. The family's problem is not improving or is worsening

2. The family withdraws prematurely from treatment

3. One or more family members refuse to attend meetings
    with the doctor

4. The doctor has difficulty bringing himself to meet
    with the family when indicated

5. The physician finds it difficult to understand the
    family's behavior

The physician should <u>refer the patient to a psychiatrist</u> if:

1. The doctor does not wish to work with the family

2. The doctor does not like the family

3. A danger of suicide or homicide in any family member exists

4. Child abuse, incest, or spouse abuse is present

5. A family member is psychotic or has a severe behavioral disturbance

6. The family problem is unusually complex

REFERENCES

Brulun JG: Effects of chronic disease on the family. J Fam Pract
    1977; 4:1057

Dubovsky S: Psychotherapeutics in Primary Care. New York, Grune &
    Stratton, 1981. pp 40-43, 183-210

Foley V: An introduction to family therapy. Family Process.
    1973; 12:179

Sackin HD, Raffe IH: Multi-problem families. Clin Soc Work
    1976; 4:34

Solomon M: A developmental, conceptual premise for family therapy.
    Family Process 1973;12:179

Solomon M: Typologies of homeostasis and their implications in
    diagnosis and treatment of the family. Family Therapy 1974;1:9

Chapter Eight
SEXUAL DYSFUNCTION

by Daniel Hoffman, M.D.

Educating couples with sexual dysfunction forms the cornerstone of many sexual therapies. An understanding of sexual physiology begins with an understanding of the four stages of sexual arousal:

1. Excitement is characterized by the development of pleasurable and erotic feelings. Respiration, heart rate and blood pressure increase, and there is a concomitant flushing of the skin. Erection occurs when the corpora cavernosa and corpus spongiosum distend with blood, under the influence of the parasympathetic nervous system. While this response is involuntary and cannot be willed, pleasurable sexual fantasies aid in the attainment of an erection.

   In the female, the breasts swell and the nipples become erect, and the clitoris also may become erect. The inner two-thirds of the vagina and the uterus begin to enlarge and the cervix begins to elevate in order to prepare for acceptance of the penis. Vasocongestion of the external genitals begins the lubrication process. The major and minor labia engorge with blood, increasing in size and extending outward, to prepare an opening for the penis. While these changes begin within 15 to 30 seconds of stimulation, it may take some time before the lubricant seeps out of the vagina and is felt on the external genitalia.

2. The plateau stage is characterized by an intensification of the changes experienced during excitement. In the male, the penis becomes filled to capacity with blood and is at its maximum size. It is not unusual for some amount of seminal fluid to seep out of the penis at this time, making pregnancy possible before ejaculation.

In the woman, the outer third of the vagina begins
to enlarge as the swelling of the labia minora increases.
The breasts continue to grow in size, and the area
around the nipples enlarges so as to engulf them,
sometimes causing the nipples to appear not to be
erect. The clitoris begins to retract underneath
its hood, and its multiple nerve endings are no
longer directly exposed to stimulation.

3. During male orgasm, heart rate and blood pressure
    continue to rise, and there may be spastic contractions
    of the extremities, with involuntary thrusting of
    the pelvis. Just before orgasm, the moment of
    ejaculatory inevitability is reached. This is the
    point beyond which ejaculation cannot be prevented.
    During ejaculation, the urethra contracts in
    rhythmic spurts every 0.8 seconds, expelling seminal
    fluid. Following orgasm, the penis is unable to regain
    its erect status for varying amounts of time, despite
    further stimulation (refractory period).

    In the female, orgasm occurs through stimulation of
    the clitoris directly (manually or orally) or
    indirectly (thrusting of the penis inside the vagina
    may cause the labia to stimulate the clitoris). Sixty
    to seventy percent of women are unable to reach orgasm
    regularly through intercourse alone and need some
    form of direct clitoral stimulation in order to climax.
    During orgasm, the uterus undergoes contractions which
    may be experienced as a pleasurable abdominal sensation.
    Many women are able to have multiple orgasms if
    further stimulation is provided.

4. Resolution is characterized by a return to preexcitement
    physiology. Heart rate, blood pressure and respiration
    become normal. The penis immediately decreases to
    one half of its erect size, and is back to normal size
    within an hour.

    In the woman, breast size returns to normal in 5 to 10
    minutes. The nipples may appear to become erect again
    as breast engorgement decreases. The clitoris returns
    to its normal size within 10 seconds after orgasm,
    the labia slowly return to their resting position and
    the vagina gradually collapses. A region of the vagina

near the cervix, which is in direct contact with
the still open cervical os, forms a cavity in which
a pool of semen collects. As the cervix descends
back to its normal resting state, it dips into the
seminal pool, maximizing the chances of fertilization.

The pattern of sexual arousal begins to change after age 50:

1. Excitement is a slower process. Men take a longer time
    to attain erection, and prolonged direct genital
    stimulation may be required. Erections may not reach
    the same firmness or fullness as in the younger man,
    and there is a decreased demand to achieve orgasm.
    Women, too, take longer to become aroused, and there
    is a significant delay in lubrication. The vagina loses
    much of its elasticity, making expansion more difficult.

2. Plateau in the elderly male lasts longer, allowing for
    better control of ejaculation. For the female over 50,
    there is less swelling of the labia, which may hang
    in limp folds. The experience of pleasurable sensation
    does not decrease with age in either sex.

3. Orgasm is shorter in both men and women. Many older
    men lose the sensation of ejaculatory inevitability,
    and the explosive force of seminal fluid is decreased.
    Older women experience fewer uterine contractions.

4. Resolution in the elderly man is accompanied by a
    more rapid loss of erection after ejaculation, and
    he experiences a longer refractory period. The
    older woman, too, experiences a more rapid return
    to the resting state.

Many people experience transient sexual problems at some time.
For example, a man who is intoxicated while attempting to have intercourse may be unable to get an erection; or, if a couple attempts to
make love when they are rushed, the man may experience a rapid (premature) ejaculation, and the woman may be unable to reach an orgasm.
Following such experiences some people begin to worry excessively about
their ability to perform the next time they have sex. This performance
anxiety distracts from the pleasurable aspects of sex, making it
difficult to maintain an erection, experience an orgasm, or otherwise
perform adequately. Subsequent failures then create still more
performance anxiety. This vicious circle, which is responsible for

many cases of acute sexual dysfunction, is easily treatable if caught early. If untreated, chronic difficulties that are more refractory to treatment may result.

Another common source of transient sexual difficulties is misunderstanding of the role of fantasy in normal sex. By providing a means through which a person may make his own sexual experience more exciting, fantasy provides increased gratification. If an individual has been taught that sexual fantasies are wrong or a sign of infidelity, his attempts to inhibit them may lead to frustration, a chronic sense of guilt, and anger at his spouse, expressed as sexual dysfunction.

The workup of a patient with a sexual dysfunction includes the following steps:

1. Obtain the information that a sexual problem is present

2. Determine whether the disorder is psychogenic or secondary to organic factors

3. Determine whether the disorder is best treated by the primary physician or by a specialist

Patients with sexual dysfunction may present to their physicians with almost any complaint, from aches and pains to depression, hoping that the doctor will ask them about their sexual functioning. Often, all that is needed to elicit a history of a sexual problem is to include a few questions about this topic in the review of systems. For example, if the doctor's suspicion has not already been aroused during the initial examination, a general question such as "how are things going at home?", followed by, "and how are things sexually between you and your spouse?" may result in the patient's telling the doctor about a sexual problem.

The most important factor in the successful treatment of sexual dysfunctions is the doctor's comfort and openness. Four useful principles of treatment are:

1. Sexual problems occur between individuals: involve both partners in treatment whenever possible

2. Educate the patient about normal sexual function, while correcting misconceptions and relieving guilt about habits (e.g., fantasizing during sex) that are not abnormal

3. Treat <u>performance anxiety</u>

4. Pay attention to <u>alterations normal in sexual</u>
   physiology, especially in older patients

CLUES TO THE DIAGNOSIS OF SEXUAL DYSFUNCTION

Embarrassment may cause some patients to avoid bringing their sexual problems to the physician's attention, while others may fear that the clinician will not feel comfortable or will think them disgusting or laughable. It is therefore important to remain alert to subtle clues that sexual dysfunction may be present and to ask about possible problems in a direct and reassuring manner. Some clues are:

1. Any marital problem

2. Insomnia

3. Chronic somatic complaints

4. Depression

5. Persistent irritation with others

6. Alcoholism or drug abuse

7. Requests of a spouse to meet with the physician
   without the knowledge of the other spouse

ENCOUNTER WITH A TYPICAL PATIENT

Mr. I. is a 42-year-old married man who complains of headaches that are worse in the evening. Physical and neurological exams are negative, and additional tests are within normal limits. The physician prescribes an analgesic and diazepam for tension headaches and sees the patient for followup one month later. When he returns, the patient appears more anxious, and the doctor decides to examine important areas of psychosocial functioning:

Dr: Tell me, Mr. I, how have things been going lately?

Pt: Oh, fine.

Dr: Have you changed jobs or experienced any problems at work?

Pt: No. As a matter of fact, I was recently promoted to supervisor.

Dr: Congratulations. How are things at home?

Pt: OK. No real problems. Both kids are in school now.

Dr: How are you and your wife getting along?

Pt: You know how married people are--every couple has its problems.

Dr: What problems do the two of you have?

Pt: Well, our personal life isn't always what it should be.

Dr: Do you mean that there's been a change in your sexual relationship?

Pt: Well, now that you ask, I have been a little worried lately. One night about a month ago I had a little too much to drink with the guys after work. I got home about 10:00 in the evening and my wife was upset with me. I was feeling, you know, in the mood, so I took her to the bedroom, and we began making love. Well, wouldn't you know it, no sooner was I ready to enter her when I lost my erection. I haven't really been able to get one since.

THE PHYSICIAN'S REACTION TO HIS PATIENT

Physicians are no less likely than their patients to have strong feelings about discussing sexual matters. If the physician is aware of his own discomfort, he can prevent it from impairing his ability to encourage openness in his patient. Common reactions are described below, with comments elucidating the information that can be obtained from them.

Physician's Reaction	*Comment*
Discomfort and embarrassment	Until the doctor gains experience in talking to his patients about sex, the social taboos against discussing sexual issues openly may make the conversation uncomfortable for him
Disgust	An extreme reaction to a patient's sexual problems may indicate a strict moral upbringing, or a sexual problem, in the doctor
Identification with the patient (the patient's problem reminds the doctor of his own)	Since most people experience transient sexual difficulties at some time, doctors may feel that they have had the same sexual problems as their patients. This identification may obscure the fact that the patient's problem usually is more severe than the doctor's
Helplessness	If the patient communicates his sense of physical impotency to the doctor, the physician may end up feeling impotent, too. He then may attempt to alleviate his feeling of helplessness by reassuring the patient prematurely
Conviction that a discussion of sexual problems does not belong in the physician's office	While moral prohibitions against sexual issues may preclude the physician's discussing them, discomfort and helplessness are more likely to contribute to this attitude

COMMON UNSUCCESSFUL APPROACHES

Doctors' approaches to sexual problems often are motivated by a wish to decrease their own, as well as their patients', anxiety. Common unsuccessful approaches are listed in the left-hand column below, followed by the patient's likely response and an explanation of the patient's behavior.

Physician's Approach	*Patient's Response*	*Explanation*
Reassure the patient that he has nothing to worry about or that the problem will resolve spontaneously	The patient says that the doctor is probably right and that it was silly to mention the problem. His impotency worsens, but he does not discuss it further	When the doctor, who represents authority, expertise, and openness, does not seem willing to discuss the patient's sexual problem, the patient feels embarrassed and experiences a lowering of his self-confidence, including his confidence in his ability to perform sexually
Tell the patient to go home and practice with his wife	The patient agrees to try, but does not approach his partner. Or, he tries harder to perform that night, and is impotent again. The next night he has a drink to bolster his	The patient is afraid that he will not be able to get an erection, and he avoids his partner. If he does try to practice, most of his attention is occupied by the question of whether he will be able to perform this time. This reinforces the cycle of performance anxiety leading to increasing sexual dysfunction that was already present when the patient first consulted the doctor

Physician's Approach	*Patient's Response*	*Explanation*
	self-confidence; the alcohol makes it difficult to get an erection, and his problem worsens	
Instruct the patient to read pornographic literature at home	The patient stops at the drugstore on the way home and buys several magazines and books. When he reads them, he becomes sexually aroused, but he fails again with his partner	There is nothing wrong with the patient's sexual interest, only his ability to translate it into action with a partner. If the patient is stimulated sexually and tries too hard to perform, the resulting performance anxiety may result in his experiencing another episode of impotency
Tell the patient that unless he stops worrying about getting an erection, he will become impotent	Performance anxiety and resulting impotency increase	The patient now worries that he may not be able to stop worrying. This causes increased concern about his problem and increased performance anxiety

A SUCCESSFUL APPROACH

The first step in treating sexual dysfunctions is to take an adequate history. After establishing that a sexual problem exists, the next step is to define the problem further:

Dr: Has this type of problem ever occurred before?

Pt: No. I've always been able to do my part.

Dr: Are you able to get an erection during the day, or when fantasizing about sex?

Pt: Yes. That's what's so frustrating. I even wake up with an erection in the morning; but I can't seem to make use of it with my wife.

Dr: Does an erection begin and then recede, or are you unable to get one when you first start to have sex?

Pt: I start with an erection, and then lose it when I try to enter my wife.

Dr: What goes through your mind at that point?

Pt: I start worrying whether I'll be able to finish the the job, or whether I'll be impotent again.

Dr: And that's when you begin to get small?

Pt: Exactly!

Dr: How is your wife responding to this?

Pt: Well, I imagine she's pretty disgusted with me.

Dr: Has she said or done anything to indicate that she is disgusted?

Pt: No. In fact, she has been very understanding, telling me not to worry.

Dr: It sounds like you may be disgusted with yourself.

Having determined that the problem is acute and reactive, the physician may make it seem less frightening and overwhelming by explaining it to the patient:

Dr: You know, Mr. I, it is not at all uncommon for alcohol to increase sexual desire while decreasing performance. The amount you had to drink that night made it physically difficult to get an erection. Since that time, your worrying that the problem might recur has interfered with your enjoyment of sex, making maintaining an erection difficult.

Pt: Does that mean I'm becoming impotent?

Dr: I think that we've caught the problem early enough. I'll work with you to see that it doesn't become chronic. The first thing I'd like to do is have your wife join us next time.

Pt: That sounds good. How soon can we meet?

The physician's matter-of-fact approach communicates that there is no reason to feel ashamed or inhibited. He then reassures the patient appropriately and makes plans to include the patient's partner in a treatment program that begins quickly.

Before proceeding with treatment, a <u>detailed sexual history</u> should be obtained. Although an initial history may be taken from each partner separately, both should be involved in evaluation and treatment planning as quickly as possible. The following information should be obtained:

1. Nature of the problem

2. Duration of the problem

3. Circumstances under which the problem began

4. Circumstances under which the problem now occurs (e.g., a problem that occurs with one partner but not another is likely to be caused by psychological, rather than organic, factors)

5. Presence of acute psychological stresses

6. Nature and duration of the relationship

7. Other stresses on the relationship

8. Partner's response to the problem

9. Changes in the relationship caused by the problem

10. Description of a typical sexual session including:

    - type and duration of foreplay

    - length of time it takes the man to ejaculate
      after entering the female

    - how often and with what type of stimulation
      the woman reaches an orgasm

11. Frequency of intercourse

12. Factual knowledge about sex

13. Attitudes toward sex of patient and partner,
    especially religious and moral taboos

14. Use of birth control

15. Drug and alcohol abuse

16. Physical health

17. Use of medications

18. Past psychiatric history

Next, the physician should decide whether the sexual problem is
likely to have an organic etiology. This is particularly important in
view of recent evidence, for example, that as many as 40-45% of cases of
erectile dysfunction (as opposed to previous estimates of 10%) are due
to physical causes. Impotence that is not organic in origin is associated with early morning erections, erections when masturbating or with
another partner, and positive nocturnal penile tumescence. The clinician
then can determine if the problem is acute, recurrent, or chronic, the
extent to which the partner is a source of support or contributes to the
problem and the influence of long-standing personality and marital
problems on sexual functioning.

Three types of sexual disorders are easily treated in the primary physician's office: disturbances that appear acutely following a psychological stress, are due to misinformation, or require education and retraining in communication of sexual needs. For example:

1. Impotency developing in the context of a stressful situation and/or aging, in a man who has previously been potent (reactive secondary impotency) and who is not experiencing severe marital discord

2. Uncomplicated premature ejaculation, in which the patient needs to learn to control his orgasmic threshold

3. Failure to achieve orgasm appearing in the context of a stressful situation, or due to poor muscle control, in a woman who was previously orgasmic (reactive secondary orgasmic dysfunction), and who is not experiencing severe marital problems

4. Difficulty with lubrication secondary to a stressful situation or to aging

TECHNIQUES USED IN THE TREATMENT OF SEXUAL DYSFUNCTIONS

Several techniques are basic to the treatment of all dysfunctions treated by the primary physician. These include:

1. Reassurance. Hearing that his problem has occurred in other people under the circumstances experienced by the patient, along with the doctor's reassurance and confidence that the disturbance can be corrected, make the problem seem less abnormal and hopeless.

2. Education. Normal sexual anatomy and physiology are reviewed in everyday language, utilizing diagrams if necessary. Then, misconceptions about sex are corrected. For example, many people do not know that 60-70% of females do not regularly reach an orgasm from intercourse alone without direct clitoral stimulation, or that the size of a man's penis is unrelated to his partner's satisfaction.

3. Improvement of communication skills. Many patients feel obligated to know their partner's likes and dislikes without the partner's having to tell them directly. This results in neither partner really knowing how to please the other. The physician corrects this problem by working with both partners, encouraging open discussion of each other's needs.

4. Physical pleasuring sessions. In order to develop a better knowledge of the partner's sexual response and to allow the couple to enjoy each other without the pressure to perform, a temporary ban is placed on any genital contact or intercourse. The couple is instructed to touch or massage each other anywhere except the genitals. They should be nude and in comfortable surroundings. When they feel comfortable, they are instructed to proceed to genital contact. If an erection or lubrication occurs, it is enjoyed without being taken as a signal that intercourse should occur. For example, should the impotent male get an erection, there is no demand for him to use it in intercourse. Instead, the couple allows the erection to recede, then restimulating the penis to its erect state. This builds the patient's confidence that should he lose an erection, another one can be attained. These sessions are most useful in the treatment of impotence and difficulty with lubrication.

After spending some time focusing only on pleasuring, the couple is ready to proceed with intercourse. The warning that the problem may recur with the feeling of increased pressure that often accompanies intercourse helps the couple to avoid feeling too disappointed if impotence or failure to lubricate reappears. They are then instructed to avoid intercourse again, building up to it more gradually. This tactic helps the couple to gain confidence that the problem can be mastered if it is experienced again.

5. Continued interest and support. The physician remains involved to help the patient and his partner deal openly with delicate and embarrassing problems.

APPROACH TO MANAGEMENT

Management of all sexual disturbances that are usually treated in primary office practice employs the basic techniques described in the previous section, with additional strategies employed for particular problems. Each of these disorders is considered below:

1. Reactive secondary impotence may appear under the following conditions:

    - In the context of a recent, obvious <u>psychological stress</u>. For example, a man who recently experienced the breakup of a long-standing relationship with a woman whom he still loves may have difficulty attaining an erection with his new girlfriend

    - When an <u>older patient</u> is unaware of changes in normal sexual physiology. If the patient is not aware of the normal increase in the length of time it takes to become aroused and decrease in fullness of erections, he may assume that he is becoming impotent. This creates performance anxiety, which makes it even more difficult to attain an erection

    - Attempting to have intercourse after <u>drinking heavily</u> or taking tranquilizers or illicit <u>drugs</u>. The resulting difficulty attaining an erection can create performance anxiety, which makes getting an erection more difficult when intercourse is attempted without alcohol or drugs

    - When starting a <u>medication</u> that decreases sexual interest or potency, without being aware of the effect of the drug on sexual performance

After instituting the appropriate general measures (e.g., reassurance and education), treatment involves the institution of sensory awareness exercises. The patient is instructed that, during a pleasuring session, when he begins to worry about whether or not he will attain an erection, he is to shift his attention to the pleasurable aspects of the session. For example, the patient might be told: "When you become aware of thinking about whether or not you'll be able to perform, you might focus on the way in which your partner is massaging you, or what your partner's skin feels like under your fingertips." This shifting of attention reinforces the pleasurable aspects of lovemaking, thereby changing a state of anxiety into one of comfort. The patient can be expected to begin having erections regularly within a month.

2. Premature ejaculation may be the presenting complaint of a male patient, or his partner may complain that his erections do not last long enough to provide her with sufficient stimulation to reach orgasm. Many clinicians feel that premature ejaculation is present if the man reaches an orgasm before his partner more than 50% of the time, assuming she is capable of orgasm through intercourse. If the patient has had this problem since adolescence, it is not likely to have an organic etiology. However, if premature ejaculation appears for the first time after the patient has been functioning sexually at a consistent level for a long time, disease of the urethra, prostate, or CNS should be considered.

Treatment of uncomplicated premature ejaculation carries an extremely high (90%) success rate. One of two techniques is utilized, depending on the couple's preference:

- In the start-stop technique, the patient masturbates to the point of ejaculatory inevitability (the point beyond which ejaculation cannot be prevented), and then ceases all stimulation. After 30-60 seconds, or when his erection is halfway back to its flaccid state, he resumes stimulation. This procedure is repeated 4-5 times per session. After the patient has practiced on his own, his partner is asked to provide the stimulation during pleasuring sessions, and the patient signals her to stop when he reaches the point

of ejaculatory inevitability. After the
couple feels comfortable with this technique,
intercourse is attempted, using the female
superior position. The man lies still,
controlling thrusting with his hands on his
partner's hips, and the couple stops thrusting at the point of ejaculatory inevitability.
Control over ejaculation should be achieved
after a maximum of one year.

- The squeeze technique also requires that the
man practice on his own before proceeding to
intercourse. When he has had sufficient
practice, he signals to his partner during
intercourse in the female superior position
that he has reached the point of ejaculatory
inevitability. She then removes his penis
from her vagina and takes it in her hand.
She places her thumb on the ventral surface
of the frenulum and her first and second
fingers on the dorsal surface, with one finger
above, and one finger below the coronal ridge.
Placing the corresponding fingers of her other
hand on top of her first hand, she exerts
strong constant pressure until he begins to
lose his erection. Intercourse is then resumed
and the procedure is repeated.

3. Reactive secondary orgasmic dysfunction has two common
modes or presentation:

- Some women who are able to reach orgasm with
masturbation, manual stimulation or oral sex
but not with intercourse feel that they are
dysfunctional, especially if their partner
tells them that they should be able to climax
through intercourse alone

- Other women may have been able to reach orgasm
with one partner, but are unable to climax with
their current partners

Essential to the treatment of reactive secondary
orgasmic dysfunction is the determination of those
circumstances under which the patient is orgasmic. A
history of previous sexual experiences will help to

determine if the patient ever has been orgasmic with
intercourse alone. A discussion of the couple's
sexual technique will determine whether they spend
enough time in foreplay or intercourse to allow
the woman a chance to reach an orgasm.

A woman who previously has been orgasmic with
intercourse, and who is not experiencing serious
conflicts in her relationships with her partner, may
benefit from an open discussion with him of their
sexual likes and dislikes. For example, a woman may
be encouraged to tell her partner that she is non-
orgasmic because he does not provide her with sufficient
clitoral stimulation. Women who are only able to reach
orgasm with direct clitoral stimulation, and their
partners, can be taught to accept this fact, not to
see it as a failing of either person, and to adjust
their sex life around it. Attention to clitoral
stimulation during foreplay and intercourse can then
make sex gratifying for both partners. Some people
have the notion that the only "good" orgasm is one which
occurs through intercourse alone; this myth should
be dispelled.

All patients with orgasmic dysfunction should be
examined for lax pubococcygeal muscles. Women whose
inability to reach orgasm is secondary to this condition
will benefit from exercises that strengthen the pubococcygeal muscles. The patient is told that the muscles
to be strengthened stop the flow of urine or close the
rectal sphincter after a bowel movement. The exercise
can be performed anywhere, anytime, with the patient
sitting or standing. It consists of contracting these
muscles, as if the patient were controlling the urine
stream, ten times in a row, three to six times a day,
for from one to four months. Strengthening these muscles
allows the patient to create more friction and clitoral
stimulation during intercourse.

4.   Difficulty with lubrication usually is seen in older
women, or in women who find it difficult to enjoy sex.
It may present as soreness when intercourse is initiated.

The treatment of this problem in younger women is similar
to the treatment of impotence in men. In addition to
general measures, sensory awareness exercises are combined

with pleasuring sessions aimed at shifting the
patient's attention away from the anxiety surrounding
whether she will be able to lubricate, and focusing
on the pleasures associated with physical contact.

Older women may not be aware that lubrication naturally
takes longer with aging. The performance anxiety
that may result from the patient's fear that she is
losing her ability to become aroused can be decreased
by explaining the normal changes in sexual physiology
that occur with aging. Sterile lubricant jellies or
vaginal estrogen creams may be prescribed to compensate
for decreased ability to lubricate.

SEXUAL DYSFUNCTIONS THAT ARE TREATED BY THE SPECIALIST

Sexual dysfunctions that are influenced by complex psychological
problems usually are treated by psychiatrists, urologists and gyne-
cologists. These include:

1. Inability to reach an orgasm. 60-70% of normal women
   are unable to reach orgasm regularly through intercourse
   alone, although most are orgasmic through oral or
   manual stimulation. Therefore, to be non-orgasmic without direct clitoral stimulation is not necessarily
   a dysfunction. Primary orgasmic dysfunction occurs in
   women who have never reached orgasm under any
   circumstances. The woman who currently is unable to
   reach orgasm but has, at some time, through some means,
   been able to climax, is said to have secondary orgasmic
   dysfunction. Reactive secondary orgasmic dysfunction
   usually is caused by misconceptions about normal sexual
   response or by a problem in sexual technique (e.g., not
   enough clitoral stimulation during foreplay or intercourse, or premature ejaculation in the partner). Other
   forms of secondary orgasmic dysfunction usually are
   caused by emotional conflicts about enjoying sex or by
   conflicts with the partner. Occasionally, physical
   disorders such as clitoral adhesions or weak pubococcygeal
   muscles are to blame, and careful gynecological examination
   is warranted for all women with orgasmic dysfunction.
   Surprisingly, the prognosis with treatment is better in
   primary than in secondary orgasmic dysfunction.

2. Sexual aversion (Frigidity). Frigidity refers to
    sexual coldness toward men, with little or no
    erotic pleasure being experienced with them, in
    women who are not homosexual. It usually is
    accompanied by an absence of vaginal vasocongestion,
    resulting in little or no lubrication during the
    excitement phase. It often is due to deep psychological
    conflicts, and has been treated with varying success
    with behavior therapy and psychoanalysis.

3. Vaginismus. Vaginismus is characterized by spasms of
    the vaginal muscles causing the vaginal entroitus to
    "snap shut" whenever the penis attempts to enter, making
    intercourse virtually impossible. It may be due to
    conflicts about sex. Prognosis with behavior therapy
    is excellent (over 80% of women are cured).

4. Erectile dysfunction (Impotency). Any problem
    characterized by interference with the ability to
    achieve or maintain an erection is an erectile
    dysfunction. If an individual never has had an erection
    with a sexual partner but is able to attain one at
    other times, such as during masturbation, he is said
    to suffer from primary impotency. If he has been able,
    on at least one occasion, to attain an erection with a
    sexual partner, he is said to suffer from secondary
    impotency. If a man has never had an erection under
    any circumstances, a physical disturbance should be
    sought. Men who get erections at some times, (e.g.,
    early in the morning or while dreaming), but not with
    their partner, are likely to have a psychogenic problem.
    All forms of secondary impotence are associated with
    performance anxiety, which often is compounded by
    problems in the relationship with the partner, and
    conflicts in the patient over sexuality. Prognosis
    with treatment is better for secondary than for primary
    impotency.

5. Retarded ejaculation. Retarded ejaculation is an
    uncommon dysfunction in which the ejaculatory reflex
    is inhibited. It may occur with only one, or with all
    partners. The patient usually has more difficulty with
    ejaculation inside than outside the vagina. Few physiologic
    causes have been described for this condition. Cure rate
    approximates 60%.

6. <u>Dyspareunia</u>. Pain on intercourse occurs in both women and men. It often is due to a combination of medical and psychological problems. Urological or gynecological examination is mandatory for patients with this complaint.

7. <u>Drive inhibition</u>. This recently described problem occurs in patients who have a conscious desire for sex but unconsciously fear it. Although they are aroused when sexual impulses cannot be acted upon (e.g., on the telephone), these patients lose interest in sex when confronted with the opportunity for physical intimacy. A variation of this problem occurs in patients who lose interest sexually in a spouse to whom they are emotionally attached while experiencing intense arousal with a relative stranger. Deep-seated fears of the dangers of sex with a loved one, depression, anxiety, anger at the spouse, some medications, and chronic illness may produce drive inhibition. When the latter problems are not present, intensive psychotherapy or sex therapy are applied, depending on whether the sexual dysfunction occurs along with other personality problems or is the only complaint.

APPROACH TO MEDICATIONS

Many medications affect sexual performance. Common alterations in sexual function are listed in the left-hand column below. The right-hand column lists classes of medication that can produce the change in function.

Alteration in Sexual Function	*Class of Drug That Produces Altered Function*
Decreased sexual responsiveness and interest (loss of libido)	Sedative-hypnotics (e.g., barbiturates); analgesics (especially narcotics); anti-androgens; adrenal steroids; chronic use of stimulants (e.g., amphetamines, cocaine) and hallucinogens; alcohol

Alteration in Sexual Function	*Class of Drug That Produces Altered Function*
Impotence	Anticholinergic drugs (e.g., atropine, probanthine); anti-androgens, some anti-hypertensives (especially quanethidine, rauwolfia alkaloids, and methyldopa); antipsychotic drugs (especially thiori-dazine and haloperidol); alcohol; tranquilizers
Increased libido	Hormones, (especially androgens); L-dopa, acute use of stimulants (amphetamines and cocaine); hallucinogens (e.g., marijuana, LSD)
Retrograde ejaculation	Phenothiazines (especially thioridazine)
Retarded ejaculation	Butyrophenones (especially haloperidol)

DIFFERENTIAL DIAGNOSIS

Because of the large number of illnesses that can cause sexual dysfunction, it is wise to rule out organic disorders before attributing any dysfunction to psychological factors. Systemic illnesses that predictably produce disturbances in sexual function include:

1. Alcohol and drug abuse

2. Venereal disease

3. Thyroid dysfunction

4. Diabetes mellitus

5. Multiple sclerosis

6. Spinal cord disease

7. Hypertension

8. Arteriosclerosis (when it causes decreased penile blood flow)

9. Liver disease, causing increased estrogen (or decreased androgen) levels

10. Peripheral neuropathy

11. Brain disease

12. Any disease debilitating or painful enough to affect sexual performance or interest

In addition, many genital and rectal disorders can affect sexual performance. These include:

1. Prostate disease

2. Lesions of the glans or foreskin of the penis

3. Varicocele

4. Hydrocele

5. Peyrones' disease

6. Lesions of the vulva, entroitus, vagina, cervix, or uterus

7. Pubococcygeal muscle weakness

8. Chronic urinary tract infections

9. Chronic gynecological infections

Loss of sexual desire also may be a presenting complaint of some psychiatric conditions, especially depression and anxiety.

USE OF THE PSYCHIATRIST

While many early and uncomplicated sexual dysfunctions can be treated by the primary physician in his office, the psychiatrist is useful in a number of ways:

The physician should consult with the psychiatrist if:

1. The etiology of the disorder is in doubt

2. The physician needs help devising a treatment plan

3. The extent to which psychological factors influence the disorder needs clarification

4. Evaluation is needed of conflicts in the relationship with the partner

5. The extent to which an illness or necessary medication is contributing to sexual dysfunction needs evaluation

The physician should refer the patient to the psychiatrist if:

1. Either partner has a severe psychiatric disorder (e.g., psychosis)

2. Severe discord in the relationship is present

3. One of the partners refuses to participate in treatment

4. One or both of the partners is involved in an extramarital affair

5. A combination of dysfunctions (e.g., impotence and premature ejaculation) is present

6. Either partner has a sexual perversion

7. Intensive long-term psychotherapy is indicated

8. The physician's treatment is not effective

9. The physician prefers not to treat sexual
    dysfunction

REFERENCES

Kaplan HS: Disorders of Sexual Desire. New York, Brunner Mazel, 1979

Kaplan HS: The New Sex Therapy. New York, Brunner Mazel, 1974

Lobitz WC: Clinical Recognition and Treatment of Sexual Dysfunctions
    In: Cozzetto F, Brettell HR: Topics in Family Practice. Miami,
    Symposium Specialists, 1976

Masters W, Johnson V: Human Sexual Inadequacy. Boston, Little Brown,
    1970

Munjack D, Oziel LJ: Evaluating Sexual Problems in Office Practice.
    Medical Aspects of Human Sexuality. 1977; 11:92

Chapter Nine
SCHIZOPHRENIA

Schizophrenia comprises a group of disorders that often begin in adolescence or early adulthood characterized by recurrent or chronic psychoses and progressive deterioration in functioning. Although some schizophrenics appear well adjusted between episodes of psychoses, they usually demonstrate some continuing maladjustment. Because they are likely not to care for themselves and because early signs of physical disease are likely to be overshadowed by psychiatric symptoms, schizophrenic patients (about 1% of the general population) are over-represented among the medically ill and die earlier than nonschizophrenic individuals. Many schizophrenics are treated for intercurrent illnesses, as well as for their psychoses, by primary care physicians.

An important contribution to the diagnosis of schizophrenic psychoses has been the elucidation by Schneider of the first-rank symptoms. These are a number of specific hallucinations and delusions, the presence of any one of which, in the absence of an organic brain disorder, strongly suggests that a schizophrenic psychosis is present.

Hallucinations include:

1. Voices speaking the patient's thoughts out loud

2. Two or more voices arguing about the patient

3. Voices commenting on the patient's actions in the third person

Delusions include the conviction that:

1. The patient's will has been taken over by an outside force, so that emotions, thoughts, impulses or actions are no longer his own (delusions of control)

2. Thoughts are being put into the patient's mind (thought insertion)

3. Thoughts are being removed from the patient's mind (thought withdrawal)

4. Thoughts are escaping from the patient's head
   so that others can hear them (thought broadcasting)

5. Bodily sensations are being imposed on the patient
   by an outside source

6. A common event has a special idiosyncratic meaning
   (delusional perceptions), e.g., a rainstorm might
   signify a message from beings from another world

The new edition of the official psychiatric nomenclature (DSM-3)
has attempted to synthesize a number of diagnostic schemes by
establishing the following criteria for a diagnosis of schizophrenia:

1. Symptom duration of at least six months. Schizophrenia-
   like illnesses lasting less than six months but more than
   two weeks are termed schizophreniform disorders, and
   those lasting less than two weeks are called brief
   reactive psychoses. Both of the latter disturbances
   occur in the context of an obvious psychosocial stress
   and are accompanied by more vivid emotional expression--
   especially fear, anger, anxiety and depression--than
   schizophrenia. They may be related to affective disorders
   and borderline syndromes, respectively.

2. Onset before age 45.

3. Deterioration in work, social relations or self-care.

4. Psychotic symptoms at some time during the course of the
   illness, especially:

   a. bizarre, absurd delusions (e.g. Schneiderian
      delusions) that are not determined by cultural
      factors

   b. delusions of persecution or jealously that are
      accompanied by any type of hallucination

   c. in the absence of hallucinations, somatic,
      grandiose, religious or other delusions
      that are not persecutory or jealous

   d. Schneiderian hallucinations

   e. hallucinations that are not consistent
      with an elated or depressed mood

5. Bizarre, idiosyncratic (autistic) thinking,
   in which ordinary logical connections between
   thoughts are replaced by associations that make
   sense only to the patient (loose associations),
   thoughts are temporarily interrupted for no
   apparent reason (blocking), and ordinary rules
   of logic do not apply (dereistic thinking).
   The patient is very difficult to understand
   and his speech may demonstrate incoherence and
   neologisms (nonsense words coined by the patient).

6. Disordered emotional expression, consisting of
   affect that is inappropriate to the content of
   the patient's thinking or that is blunted
   (reduced in emotional expression) or flattened
   (without emotional expression).

7. Grossly disorganized behavior or a decrease in
   spontaneous, goal-directed activity.

8. Symptoms are not caused by an organic brain syndrome.

CLUES TO THE DIAGNOSIS OF SCHIZOPHRENIA

1. Withdrawal from social interactions

2. Bizarre, idiosyncratic thinking

3. Peculiar behavior

4. Incoherent speech

5. Blunted, flat or inappropriate affect

6. Hallucinations or delusions, especially if bizarre
   and if unrelated to a depressed or elated mood

7. Confusion about identity or the meaning of life

8. Preoccupation with vague philosophical or
   political ideas

9. Reports of strange or unusual experiences
   (e.g. contact with the dead or sensing the
   presence of a powerful but unknown force)

10. First onset of psychotic symptoms in the late
    teens or twenties

11. Pronounced ambivalence that makes it difficult to initiate meaningful action

12. Severe hypochondriacal preoccupations

13. Feelings of not being real

14. Past history of schizophrenia

15. Family history of schizophrenia

16. Absence of signs of OBS

17. Negative drug or alcohol history

18. Feeling of great emotional distance from the interviewer

ENCOUNTER WITH A TYPICAL PATIENT

Miss S is a 48 year-old-woman who has made an appointment in the outpatient department because of stomach pain. She appears for her visit dressed in an old baggy cloth coat and a ragged sweater, glaring anxiously around the waiting room. During the past twenty-five years she has had an unknown number of psychiatric hospitalizations, after each one of which she was lost to follow-up. She has a large medical chart that reveals numerous brief hospitalizations and failed outpatient appointments for a variety of complaints. Following her most recent hospitalization, she was to be followed at a local mental health center. However, instead of keeping her appointment, she discontinued her medication and began attending medical clinics, complaining of gastrointestinal, cardiac and pulmonary symptoms. Her current visit begins with the following conversation:

Dr: What seems to be wrong?

Pt: I have this pain in my stomach...I'm sure it's my gallbladder. I need x-rays. Would you like a cigarette?

Dr: No thanks, I don't smoke. How do you know it's your gallbladder?

Pt: I know it is. The pain starts here (pointing to her abdomen). Are you sure you don't smoke? And the pain moves here (points to her back and lifts the back of her coat and dress).

Dr: O.K., you don't have to get undressed yet.

Pt: The pains are really there, doctor. They're
     killing me. They're all killing me. You know
     how the pains come and go? I know there's a
     purpose to it. The gallbladder is the seat
     of such pain.

Dr: Who's killing you?

Pt: You know. If you'll only take out my gallbladder
     it'll be alright.

THE PHYSICIAN'S REACTION TO HIS PATIENT

Schizophrenic patients often evoke reactions in their physicians
which, while disturbing, may suggest the diagnosis. The right hand
column below offers comments on some common reactions to schizophrenic
patients.

Physician's Reaction	*Comment*
Inability to understand what the patient is talking about	If the doctor is not preoccupied with personal concerns, failure to understand a patient may indicate that the patient's speech is unintelligible due to loose associations and idiosyncratic logic
Conviction that the patient is simulating her symptoms	If the patient's bizarre logic and behavior make the physician anxious, he may attempt to minimize her symptoms, and hence the necessity of his having to work with her, by assuming that they are under her conscious control
Feeling that the patient is a weird, bizarre person	Because the patient is emotionally distant from other people, it is difficult to empathize with her distress

Physician's Reaction	*Comment*
Conclusion that all of the patient's physical complaints are symptoms of her psychosis	In addition to suffering from somatic delusions and hallucinations, schizophrenics often interpret physical illness in an idiosyncratic way, making it difficult to distinguish organic disease from the patient's fabrications
Conviction that the patient is hopelessly psychotic	The bizarre logic, hallucinations, delusions, and loss of relatedness that accompany schizophrenic decompensation may be so disturbing to the physician that he ignores the fact that the patient is able to function at a higher level between psychotic episodes. This may lead to an inappropriate amount of therapeutic nihilism

COMMON UNSUCCESSFUL APPROACHES

The schizophrenic's puzzling behavior often make the physician feel unsure how to proceed with diagnosis and treatment. Common interventions are described below, along with the patient's response and an explanation of her behavior.

Physician's Approach	*Patient's Response*	*Explanation*
Tell the patient she has an emotional problem and refer her back to the mental health center	The patient does not keep her appointment, returning instead to the clinic with intensified complaints	In addition to defining her problem as a medical one, the patient already has demonstrated her unwillingness to accept psychiatric follow-up. Premature referral does not allow the patient to develop a working relationship with the physician that might facilitate appropriate treatment once organic disease is ruled out

Physician's Approach	Patient's Response	Explanation
Show the patient her x-rays or test reports to prove that she does not have gallbladder disease	The patient is convinced that the doctor is showing her the wrong x-rays	Delusions represent an attempt to restore psychological equilibrium by providing an explanation of the patient's distress that is understandable to her. Since her ideas are reassuring and understandable to her, she will attempt to defend them from attempts to prove them wrong
Reassure the patient and make a follow-up appointment in six months	The patient attends a different clinic as a new patient, and is referred back to the original physician with increased complaints	The patient is suffering from a disorganizing process that causes considerable anxiety. She reaches out to the doctor as best she can by developing physical complaints. Premature reassurance and a distant follow-up appointment sever the developing connection to the potentially helpful doctor, and increase the patient's panic
Treat the patient's gastrointestinal complaints with Maalox and her anxiety with diazepam	The patient's symptoms continue, as do her unannounced visits to the clinic	Until the proper medications are prescribed, the underlying psychosis is likely to continue. The patient does not make appointments because she is afraid that the doctor will find a way to avoid her if he expects her

A SUCCESSFUL APPROACH

An interested, non-judgmental, confident attitude in the doctor is therapeutic for even the most disturbed patient. Rather than arguing about their veracity, the physician can organize his approach around the patient's complaints:

Dr: Miss S, I know that you are frightened that there is something very wrong with you, and I will try to help you with your problem.

Pt: It's this pain. It's through my gallbladder. It's important that you believe me.

Dr: I believe that something extremely upsetting is happening; but it can be treated. Now let me examine you and order some tests.

The physician has acknowledged that a serious problem exists, without either agreeing or disagreeing with the patient's delusional ideas. He then begins to establish a working relationship with her by proceeding with the work-up in a businesslike manner, obtaining reasonable non-invasive studies, and obtaining further psychiatric history. The patient's confidence and cooperation are more likely to be obtained when she is reassured that her complaints are not being discounted. However, potentially dangerous tests that simply are not indicated should not be obtained merely to placate the patient.

CONFIRMATION OF THE DIAGNOSIS

As the doctor continues his work-up, he can proceed to confirm the diagnosis of schizophrenia, investigating first the patient's history:

1. Inquire about a <u>history of past psychotic episodes</u>. This may be introduced with the question, "Have you ever had symptoms similar to the ones you are now experiencing?" or, "Have you ever had any other unusual or disturbing experiences?"

2. Review any <u>past psychiatric hospitalization and treatment.</u> Pay attention to which treatments have been helpful, as these are likely to be helpful again.

3. Inquire about the <u>use of drugs</u> (especially amphetamines, cocaine, PCP) and <u>alcohol</u>.

4. Ask about a family history of schizophrenia.

5. Review the family history of treatment for schizophrenia.
Good response to a particular antipsychotic drug in a family member
may indicate that that person actually was schizophrenic. Also, since
familial patterns of response to antipsychotic drugs seem to exist,
good response to a particular drug in a family member may predict
good response in the patient.

During the psychological examination of the patient, the physician
should pay particular attention to the presence of the following factors:

1. Inappropriate, flat, or bizarre affect.

2. Hallucinations and delusions, especially Schneiderian first-
rank symptoms. The physician should ask about each of these, for
example, "Have you had the experience of hearing your thoughts spoken
out loud?" or, "Have you had the feeling that your will-power has been
taken over by an outside force?"

3. Unusual, idiosyncratic or disorganized thinking or speech
that is difficult to understand.

4. Abnormal interpretations of proverbs and similarities.
Schizophrenic patients, even when they are not psychotic, may demonstrate
loose associations and bizarre, autistic or concrete thinking when given
a task requiring abstract thought:

  -Abstracting ability is tested by asking the patient
   to explain the most general meaning of common proverbs.
   For example, a nonschizophrenic patient who was asked
   to explain the proverb "You can't tell a book by its
   cover" might reply: "You don't always know what people
   are like on the inside by paying attention only to
   their appearance." A schizophrenic patient may respond:
   "If you open the book of life the answer is inside"
   (idiosyncratic response) or "because it's closed"
   (concrete answer).

  -Asking the patient to tell how two items are similar
   is another test of abstracting ability that may evoke
   schizophrenic logic. For example, if a nonschizophrenic
   patient were asked what an apple and an orange had in
   common, he might reply that they are both fruit. A
   schizophrenic patient might pay attention only to one
   part of the problem that had special significance
   to him, for example, "they both have skins like worms."
   A concrete response would be: "They're both round."

5. <u>Absence of evidence of organic brain syndrome.</u> If the mental status exam reveals disorientation, memory loss, and disturbed attention and consciousness, the diagnosis of schizophrenia should be questioned. Concrete thinking may be present in organic brain syndromes as well as in schizophrenia.

6. <u>A feeling of great emotional distance</u> from the patient.

APPROACH TO PSYCHOTHERAPY

Most patients with acute schizophrenic psychoses are treated by the psychiatrist, who attempts to restore psychological equilibrium as rapidly and completely as possible. Chronic care, however, is as likely to be provided by the nonpsychiatric physician. Long-term treatment has as its goal the maintenance of the patient outside of the hospital at his highest possible level of functioning for as long as possible. To accomplish this goal, <u>supportive psychotherapy</u> is instituted. This treatment emphasizes the patient's adaptation to reality and avoids stimulating his already overactive fantasy world. The following guidelines are useful:

1. Make regular appointments which begin and end on schedule. Ten to thirty minutes every few weeks to every few months usually is sufficient

2. Prepare the patient in advance for the doctor's absences, and provide him with the name of the covering physician.

3. Begin sessions by allowing the patient to bring up any issues that might be on his mind. Then listen respectfully to his concerns, without necessarily attempting to resolve them or make the patient aware of the deeper meanings of his statements

4. Emphasize the importance of taking antipsychotic drugs regularly, exploring objections to adhering to medication schedules

5. Offer advice about everyday decisions

6. Maintain a professional demeanor and distance from the patient

7. Direct the conversation away from complex fantasies and preoccupations toward real-life events

8. Call the patient or his caretakers if he misses an appointment without calling. Missed appointments may be the first sign of impending decompensation

9. Meet the patient's family or other sources of emotional support. The physician's interventions may be necessary to prevent them from covertly encouraging the patient to discontinue his medication or to respond to their conflicts by developing psychotic symptoms

10. Maintain contact with social agencies (e.g., halfway houses, mental health centers) working with the patient. Regular, brief meetings, even on the telephone, to coordinate treatment efforts are essential when multiple caretakers are involved

11. Be alert for the presence of suicidal and homicidal thoughts. The patient is at special risk if he hears voices telling him to hurt himself or someone else (command hallucinations)

12. Relapses are common in chronic schizophrenia, and rehospitalization and an increase in medication may be necessary from time to time. These should be approached without doctor or patient feeling that they have failed. Hospitalizing a decompensating patient before he becomes completely disorganized is preferable to waiting until hospitalization can be "justified" by severe psychotic symptoms

APPROACH TO MEDICATIONS

Antipsychotic drugs (also called neuroleptics or major tranquilizers) greatly facilitate the chronic treatment of schizophrenia. They ameliorate many schizophrenic symptoms, including anxiety, agitation, hallucinations, delusions and conceptual disorganization, and generally facilitate outpatient management. Discontinuation of antipsychotic medication may result in return of symptoms within three to six months, often requiring rehospitalization. The mechanism of action of neuroleptics in controlling schizophrenic symptoms is thought to be related in part to central dopamine blockade.

The principal indication for the use of antipsychotic drugs is the treatment of acute or chronic schizophrenia. They are also useful in the treatment of acute mania, some depressions with agitation and,

in very low doses, some organic brain syndromes. Antipsychotic drugs
also are sometimes used as antiemetics, and low doses of nonsedating
neuroleptics are very occasionally used in the treatment of non-
psychotic anxiety in patients who cannot tolerate the sedation
caused by antianxiety drgus. Because of their numerous dangerous side
effects, especially those associated with long-term use, these drugs
must be clearly indicated and their potential benefits must outweigh
their many dangers, before they are prescribed.

Five major classes of antipsychotic drugs are available: phenothiazines, butyrophenones, thioxanthenes, dihydroindolones and
dibenzoxazepines. Phenothiazines and the one available butyrophenone,
haloperidol, are most commonly used in the treatment of schizophrenia.
Other classes of neuroleptics are reserved for nonresponders to
phenothiazines and haloperidol.

Some neuroleptics (e.g., chlorpromazine, thioridazine) are very
sedating, while others (e.g., haloperidol, fluphenazine) do not have
strongly sedative side effects. With the exception of thioridazine,
whose anticholinergic properties ameliorate this effect, most effective
neuroleptics produce involuntary movements (extrapyramidal or Parkin-
sonian side effects). Postural hypotension, due to alpha-adrenergic
blockade, is produced by some phenothiazines and thioxanthenes. Fatal
cardiac arrhythmias also have been reported with some antipsychotic
drugs, especially thioridazine. Because of the anticholinergic
properties of many neuroleptics, other anticholinergic drugs (e.g.,
antidepressants, antiparkinsonian drugs) should be added only with
great caution. Uses and important properties of commonly used antipsychotic drugs are summarized in the tables at the end of this
chapter.

SELECTION OF AN ANTIPSYCHOTIC DRUG

The choice of an antipsychotic drug is determined mostly by the
physician's familiarity with the medication. Additional factors to be
taken into account include:

1. A favorable or unfavorable response of the patient
    to a particular drug in the past usually predicts
    a good or bad response to that drug in the present

2. A favorable or unfavorable response to a particular
    drug in a family member may predict a similar
    response to the patient

3. Sedating neuroleptics (e.g., chlorpromazine)
    are useful for the control of anxiety or
    agitation in schizophrenic patients

4. Nonsedating antipsychotic drugs (e.g., haloperidol)
    are the drugs of first choice in patients who
    object to feeling "snowed" or sedated

5. Injectable long-acting (depot) fluphenazine
    Prolixin) and haloperidol (Haldol) are useful
    for patients who forget or are unwilling to take
    medication regularly

6. Haloperidol is safest for patients with cardio-
    vascular disease and sometimes is used to sedate
    agitated patients with organic brain disease

How to Prescribe Antipsychotic Drugs

The following guidelines apply to prescribing neuroleptics to
schizophrenic patients:

1. Begin with a test dose of 50 mg. of chlorpromazine
    p.o. or 25 mg. i.m. or its equivalent and observe
    the patient for 1-2 hours. If the patient does
    not tolerate the drug (e.g., develops severe
    orthostatic hypotension or increased psychotic
    symptoms), try a different class of neuroleptic
    (e.g., haloperidol).

2. If the patient tolerates the test dose, give 100-150
    mg. of chlorpromazine (or equivalent dose of another
    drug) daily for chronic maintenance.

3. Increase the dose by 25-50 mg. of chl. promazine
    (or equivalent dose of another drug) every two
    days until a maintenance dose of 75-400 mg./day
    (or equivalent) is reached or until the patient's
    symptoms are controlled.

4. Because of the long half-life of neuroleptics,
    the entire daily dose may be given in one or two
    doses. Taking the entire dose at night minimizes
    daytime sedation and decreases the likelihood of
    the patient's forgetting to take some of his medi-
    cation. Also, anticholinergic (dry mouth, blurred
    vision, etc.) and Parkinsonian side effects are less
    bothersome when the patient is asleep. However,
    nightmares occasionally result when large doses of
    antipsychotics are taken at night.

5. If daytime sedation is preferred, for example in an
    anxious or agitated patient, give a sedating neuro-
    leptic in divided dose during the day.

6. Acute schizophrenia is treated in a hospital with
    high doses of neuroleptics (400 mg-2 grams per day
    of chlorpromazine or equivalent). The dose is
    increased until symptoms are under control or
    side effects become intolerable. After the patient's
    condition has stabilized, the dose of medication is
    reduced and he is followed as an outpatient. Anti-
    psychotic drugs are continued for about six months
    after psychotic symptoms have remitted. The dose of
    medication is then gradually discontinued over the
    next 3-6 months. The patient is followed regularly
    to provide support and to monitor for return of
    symptoms. If psychotic symptoms begin to return
    after medication is discontinued (usually within a
    few months, but may take longer), medication is
    re-instituted and/or its dosage is increased until
    symptoms are controlled. After a few months an attempt
    is again made to withdraw the drug.

7. All patients with resolvéd acute schizophrenic
    psychoses, and most with chronic psychotic symptoms,
    should receive at least one trial off of antipsychotic
    medication. If the acutely psychotïc patient's
    symptoms do not return, or if chronic symptoms are
    no worse without medication, the drug should not be
    resumed.

8. Patients who continue to relapse or whose symptoms
    worsen without medication should be continued on
    the lowest dose of neuroleptic that will control
    their symptoms.

9. Consider providing patients receiving long-term
    maintenance therapy with one or two drug-free
    days per week or one per week per month. Such
    "drug holidays" reduce the absolute amount of
    drug ingested over time and may decrease the
    patient's chance of developing complications of
    long-term drug use, especially tardive dyskinesia
    (see p. 251).

10. Failure to take antipsychotic medication as pre-
    scribed is a common cause of relapse in chronic
    schizophrenic patients. Consider this possibility
    if the patient begins to decompensate for no
    apparent reason. If the patient is not taking his
    medication, discuss the meaning of this behavior
    with the patient and his family. For example,
    some patients may feel that they do not need to

take medication if they are not sick, others harbor delusional fears of being influenced by the drug, and a few prefer psychotic symptoms to the boredom of everyday reality.

11. If the patient still has difficulty taking his medication, consider changing the dosage schedule (e.g., decreasing the number of times the patient takes a pill each day), using a liquid concentrate (and having the patient's family observe him swallow it), changing to a medication the patient finds more tolerable, or prescribing an injectable long-acting drug every 2-3 weeks.

12. Extrapyramidal side effects usually appear shortly after the patient begins the anti-psychotic drug and subside within a few weeks. Since many patients do not develop these side effects, antiparkinsonian medications should not be prescribed unless symptoms appear. Treatment of these side effects with anti-parkinsonian drugs should be discontinued after 4 weeks-3 months.

13. Several drug interactions may be troublesome to patients taking antipsychotic drugs in a medical setting:

   a. Potentiation of sedatives and analgesics (can be useful to some patients with chronic pain)

   b. Enhancement of effects of alcohol

   c. Additive effects with other anticholinergic drugs (e.g., antidepressants, morphine)

   d. Lowering of seizure threshold

   e. Increased respiratory depression when administered with narcotic analgesics

   f. Inhibition of action of levodopa and quanethidine

   g. Severe hypotension when administered with epinephrine

   h. Enhancement of metabolism of antipsychotics by barbiturates

i. Possible enhanced CNS toxicity with lithium
    and haloperidol

j. Decreased phenothiazine levels with lithium

k. Inhibition of metabolism of both propranolol
    and chlorpromazine when administered together

PROGNOSIS

As the concept of schizophrenia continues to evolve, it is
increasingly considered to be characterized by acute exacerbations,
each of which is followed by increased residual impairment or by a
chronically downhill course. Although some experts would question
the diagnosis of schizophrenia when premorbid functioning is entirely
regained following an acute psychotic episode, considering such psychoses
to be variants of mania, the factors outlined below seem to differentiate
"good prognosis" (reactive) from "bad prognosis" (process) schizophrenia.
The latter variety is more likely to cause increasing social, behavioral
and emotional debilitation.

Factor	_Good Prognosis_	_Bad Prognosis_
age at onset	older	younger
obvious psycho-social precipitant	present	absent
premorbid adjustment	working	not working
	able to establish relationships	socially isolated
	seemingly well-adjusted	eccentric
mode of onset	sudden, with florid symptoms	gradual, with progressive with-drawal
affective symptoms	confusion; depression; mania	flat or blunted affect
family history	positive for affective disease; negative for schizophrenia	positive for schizophrenia

DIFFERENTIAL DIAGNOSIS

When a patient presents with a history of social withdrawal and bizarre thinking, displays some of the characteristic hallucinations and delusions and does not have signs of organic brain disease, the diagnosis of schizophrenia is clear. However, not all clinical pictures are this obvious. Conditions that may be confused with schizophrenia are considered below, opposite salient differentiating features from the history or examination:

Psychiatric Diagnosis	*Salient Differentiating Features*
Organic brain disease may produce psychotic symptoms that can be confused with schizophrenia. Temporal lobe lesions are notorious for producing bizarre behavior without an obvious alteration in consciousness	-Disorientation and short-term memory loss are rare in schizophrenia, and common in OBS -Hallucinations are more likely to be visual, poorly organized and accompanied by illusions in OBS, and to be auditory, complex, and well-organized in schizophrenia -Schizophrenic delusions are often more bizarre and less related to real life events than those of OBS -EEG is normal in schizophrenia, but may be abnormal in OBS
Mania may be extremely difficult to distinguish from acute schizophrenia when the patient is agitated, paranoid and difficult to understand	-The manic patient is more emotionally engaged with people in his environment -Manic flight of ideas retains the normal logical connections between ideas, although ideas shift very quickly -First-rank symptoms are absent in mania -Schizophrenic patients usually have a negative family history of mania and negative past history of a positive response to lithium or antidepressants -Recovery from acute psychosis tends to be more complete after mania

Psychiatric Diagnosis	*Salient Differentiating Features*
Depression of psychotic degree, when accompanied by delusions or hallucinations, sometimes is confused with schizophrenia, especially when the depressed patient withdraws from others and gradually ceases to function	-Depressive delusions and hallucinations usually center around sin, punishment, or bodily decary -The psychotically depressed patient has an obviously severely depressed mood -Vegetative signs are absent in schizophrenia -Family history of depression is less prominent in schizophrenia -Antidepressants often worsen schizophrenic symptoms
Alcoholic hallucinosis occurs after cessation of heavy drinking and consists of threatening auditory hallucinations with a clear sensorium. When symptoms do not clear in a few days, the patient may actually be schizophrenic	-History of recent heavy drinking or cessation of drinking -Symptoms usually clear within a few days
Amphetamine psychosis is clinically indistinguishable from paranoid schizophrenia. It occurs in patients taking more than 90 mg/day of amphetamine and lasts from 2-19 days	-History of heavy amphetamine intake exists -Recovery is rapid if the patient is denied access to the drug
Phencyclidine (PCP; Angel Dust) intoxication may produce paranoia, hallucinations, a sense of slowed time, severe anxiety and agitation, and bizarre or violent behavior, that may mimic schizophrenia	-Recent history of drug ingestion -Symptoms subside within 3-6 hours -Neurological symptoms frequently occur, especially nystagmus, ataxia, dysarthria, numbness, hypertension and diaphoresis

Psychiatric Diagnosis	*Salient Differentiating Features*
Some patients with <u>person-ality disorders</u> develop paranoid psychoses (<u>brief reactive psychoses</u>) in the context of an intense relationship, unstructured situation (e.g., psycho-therapy) or drug abuse	-Symptoms occur in the context of an intense social or psycho-therapeutic relationship -Symptoms abate within a few hours to a week or two -The patient responds immediately to structure and limit setting -Antipsychotic drugs worsen symptoms
Severe <u>obsessions</u> (e.g., in <u>obsessive-compulsive disorders</u> and obsessional concerns about health in <u>hypochondriasis</u> may at times be difficult to distinguish from delusions. In addition, schizophrenics frequently develop hypo-chondriacal preoccupations	-The obsessional patient usually is aware at some point that his worries are irrational, even if he is dominated by them -Schizophrenic thinking usually is evident on formal examination
Conscious (<u>malingering</u>) and unconscious (<u>factitious disorder</u> or <u>Ganser syndrome</u>) simulation of schizophrenia occasionally occurs in patients who wish to escape some legal sanction	-Obvious gain results from being thought insane (the patient may not admit to his legal situation initially) -Symptoms are inconsistent -Symptoms are present primarily when the patient thinks that he is being watched

USE OF THE PSYCHIATRIST

The physician should <u>consult with the psychiatrist</u>:

1. To confirm the diagnosis of schizophrenia

2. To develop a treatment plan

3. For assistance in choosing a medication
    and dosage

4. To evaluate the danger of suicide or homicide

5. If the treatment plan is unsuccessful

6. If the patient's family is having difficulty
    adjusting to his illness

7. If the physician is unable to convince the
    patient to take medication regularly

8. If psychotic symptoms do not remit

The physician should <u>refer the patient to a psychiatrist</u> if:

1. The patient develops an acute psychosis

2. A danger of suicide or homicide exists

3. An intensive psychological intervention is
    indicated

4. Intensive psychotherapy or family therapy
    is indicated

5. The physician does not wish to treat the patient

Table 8.1

PROPERTIES OF COMMONLY USED ANTIPSYCHOTIC (NEUROLEPTIC) DRUGS

Class	Examples	Relative Potency	Sedative Properties	Anticholinergic Side Effects	Usual Daily Maintenance Dose (mg.) in Chronic Care	Comments
Pheno-thiazines	-Chlorpromazine (Thorazine)	Low	Strong	Strong	75-400	-Still the best all-around antipsychotic drug
	-Thioridazine (Mellaril)	Low	Moderate	Strong	75-400	-Should not be prescribed in doses greater than 800 mg/day
	-Trifluoperazine (Stelazine) -Fluphenazine (Prolixin)	High	Weak	Moderate	4-20	-Fluphenazine is available in depot form which is injected q. 2 weeks
Butyro-phenones	-Haloperidol (Haldol)	High	Weak	Weak	5-40	-Produces minimal hypotension and may be most useful in patients with heart disease
Thiox-anthenes	-Thiothixene (Navane)	High	Weak	Moderate	20-30	-Patients who do not respond to one of the other classes or who have a past history or family history of response to one of these medications should receive a trial on these drugs
Dihydro-indolones	-Molindone (Moban)	Moderate	Moderate	High	20-100	
Diben-zoxazepines	-Loxapine (Loxitane)	Moderate	Moderate	Low	60-100	

Table 8.2

COMMON SIDE EFFECTS OF NEUROLEPTICS AND THEIR TREATMENT

Organ System	Syndrome	Manifestations	Treatment or Prevention
CNS	-Akathesia	-Motor restlessness and feeling of inability to sit still, not motivated by anxiety	Acute treatment: -p.o. or i.v. diphenhydramine (Benadryl) -intramuscular antiparkinsonian drug (e.g., benztropine, trihexyphenidyl)
	-Acute dystonia	-Acute spasm of muscles of neck, tongue, eyes or trunk	
	-Parkinsonism	-Reversible stiffness, tremor, sometimes bradykinesia	-Do not begin antiparkinsonian drugs unless these side effects appear -oral antiparkinsonian drug for 4 weeks - 3 months -decrease dose of the antipsychotic drug
	-Tardive Dyskinesia	-Dyskinesias of tongue and face, choreoathetoid movements of extremities, and abnormal movements of neck and trunk, usually but not always appearing after years of treatment following a reduction in dose -Symptoms are worsened by antiparkinsonian drugs	-No treatment known. May be prevented by prescribing the least amount of drug possible and utilizing drug-free holidays
	-Anticholinergic delirium (acute OBS)	-Psychotic symptoms -Dry skin -Hyperpyrexia -Midriasis -Tachycardia	-Discontinue drug -I.V. physostigmine for severe agitation or fever

Table 8.2 contd.

Organ System	Syndrome	Manifestations	Treatment or Prevention
Auto-nomic nervous system	-Alpha adrenergic blockade	-Orthostatic hypotension	-Advise patient to stand up slowly -Treat acute hypotension with norepinephrine, not epinephrine -Avoid beta adrenergic stimulation -Change to another medication
		-Inhibition of ejaculation	-Change to another medication
	-Cholinergic blockade	-Dry mouth, blurred vision, constipation, tachycardia	-Diabetic hard candy ameliorates dry mouth
		-Precipitation of glaucoma -Precipitation of urinary retention	-Contraindicated in patients with predisposition to glaucoma or prostrate disease
Cardio-vascular	-Cardiac toxicity	-Sudden death from cardiac arrhythmia	-EKG at regular intervals may not predict patients at risk
	-Tachycardia	-Due to anticholinergic action	-Change to another drug
Hemato-logic	-Leukopenia and agranulocytosis	-Sudden appearance within the first two months of treatment	-Advise patient to call immediately for sore throat, fever, etc., and obtain immediate blood count -Discontinue drug -Prophylactic blood counts are of no value
Eye	-Pigmentary retinopathy	-Reported with doses of thioridazine greater than 800 mg/day	-Do not exceed 800 mg/day of thioridazine
Skin	-Photosensitivity	-Easy sunburning	-Advise patient to avoid strong sunlight and use sunscreens

REFERENCES

Arieti S: Interpretation of Schizophrenia. New York, Basic Books, 1974

Camietski S, Albott W: How to Fail in the Treatment of Schizophrenic People: A Primer. Bull Menn Clinic 1976; 40:118

Davis JM: Recent Developments in the Drug Treatment of Schizophrenia. Am J Psychiatry 1976; 133:208

Orlov P, Kasparian G, DiMascio A, et al: Withdrawal of Antiparkinsonian Drugs. Arch Gen Psychiatry 1971; 25:419

Pincus JH, Tucker GJ: Behavioral Neurology (2nd Ed) Boston, Oxford University Press, 1978

Shader RI (ed): Manual of Psychiatric Therapeutics. Boston, Little Brown, 1975

Wing J, Nixon J: Discriminating Symptoms in Schizophrenia. Arch Gen Psychiatry 1975; 32:853

Chapter Ten

PSYCHIATRIC EMERGENCIES

A psychiatric emergency is an acute disturbance in behavior, feeling, or thinking that, if left unattended, can result in harm to the patient or his environment. The emergency may be identified by the patient, his family or friends, or only by his physician. There are times when, even though an emergency exists, patients give few clues to how desperate they are feeling. At these times the physician must be familiar with the characteristics of patients in crisis in order to identify the problem and to initiate treatment.

Psychiatric emergencies may manifest themselves as an impulse to hurt oneself or others (including one's children). Sometimes an emergency is created by an assault on the patient, for example, rape or spousal violence. At other times, emergencies are created by intense anxiety with resultant hyperventilation or agitation.

Emergencies develop when an internal (e.g., a psychological conflict or external (e.g., loss of health) stress overwhelms an individual's ability to cope with a problem. Coping ability may fail because of the overwhelming nature of the problem or because of the inherent weakness of the patient's defenses and resources. Often there are a number of factors present. For example, a divorce may reactivate previously unresolved grief about the earlier death of a parent and lead to suicidal behavior in a patient whose coping mechanisms (defenses) are weakened by alcohol. Psychiatric emergencies often represent maladaptive attempts to regain psychological homeostasis when no other solution to the patient's problems is apparent to him. Even suicide may seem to the patient like the only possible means of adapting to an insolvable problem.

In a potential emergency the physician has four main tasks:

1. To evaluate the potential lethality of the situation

2. To decide whether altered behavior is caused by an organic or a psychological disturbance

3. To institute emergency treatment designed to prevent a lethal outcome

4. To help the patient begin to find more adaptive solutions
    to his problems

A thorough psychological evaluation in an emergency has great
value. Patients in crisis often need the physician's objectivity to
help reduce their confusion about the nature of their problem. During
a successful evaluation, a chaotic story may become intelligible to
both patient and physician. Simply putting his thoughts in sufficient
order to describe his problem to the physician may help the patient
to feel more in control, at least of his ability to relate a history to
another person. Also, since people in crisis suffer from markedly
lowered self-esteem, a helpful and hopeful listener can help the patient
to regain lost confidence by indicating that he is not beyond help.

During the initial work-up of a psychiatric emergency, the physician
should pay attention to:

1. The observable behavior of the patient. Appearance can be
    deceiving. A calm patient may be highly suicidal, while an
    agitated patient may not be dangerous.

2. The history from the patient: Why now? Careful scrutiny
    usually reveals a precipitant of the current crisis.

3. The history from friends or relatives. Information about
    dangerousness (e.g., a threat to kill someone) may be
    volunteered by a family member or friend. This is especially
    important if the patient seems confused or withholding, or
    if the story just does not seem to make sense. If a family
    member is hesitant to speak truthfully in front of the patient,
    it is helpful to interview the family member separately.

4. The patient's resources. Friends and family may be part of
    the problem or the solution. Look for "death wishes" or
    collusion in suicide, alcoholism, child abuse, incest and
    spousal violence.

5. Past history of dangerous behavior. Patients who have been
    suicidal, assaultive, or homicidal in the past are at greater
    risk of acting this way again when they are under stress.

6. The mental status examination. A disturbance of attention,
    orientation and short-term memory suggests the presence of
    an organic brain syndrome, which may reduce the patient's
    impulse control and increase his potential dangerousness
    to himself or others   (see pp. 86-96).

7. The physical examination. Attention should be paid to signs
    of substance abuse (e.g., needle tracks), fighting (e.g.,
    broken knuckles), and suicide attempts (e.g., scars on wrists).

8. The physician's intuition. A feeling of uneasiness, anxiety, or unexplained sadness may be the doctor's only clue that an apparently calm patient is barely able to keep himself from acting on intense underlying emotions. If a physician does not "feel right" about a patient, he should not ignore this important source of information.

Following the initial evaluation the physician must answer six questions:

1. Do I appreciate the seriousness of this patient's situation or am I missing important clues to the danger he is in?

2. Has the patient relaxed and become more hopeful during the examination?

3. Has the crisis lessened or resolved, or is it unchanged?

4. Do I dare send the patient home, or am I sending him back to an environment that will provoke further decompensation?

5. If I am going to send the patient home, what kind of follow-up have I arranged? Will the patient follow the treatment plan?

6. Do I need an immediate consultation with a psychiatrist in order to help me to answer these questions?

CLUES TO THE DIAGNOSIS OF PSYCHIATRIC EMERGENCIES

1. Past history of assaultive, homicidal, suicidal or other destructive behavior

2. History of multiple accidents

3. A recent major life change (e.g., death, divorce, loss of health) or other stress

4. Significant anxiety or depression

5. A history of vague somatic complaints, doctor shopping or increased concern about health

6. History from a family member or friend of homicidal or suicidal threats

7. History of drug or alcohol abuse

8. Presence of psychotic symptoms

9. Presence of an organic brain syndrome

10. Presence of a distinctly uneasy feeling in the doctor

11. Repeated visits to different physicians or emergency rooms

THE VIOLENT PATIENT

ENCOUNTER WITH A TYPICAL PATIENT

Mr. V. is a 25-year-old unemployed steel worker brought in by the police for a scalp wound tnat he received in a barroom brawl. In the hall one of the nurses mentions that Mr. V. is notorious for starting fights. As the doctor begins to suture the patient's wound, the following interchange occurs:

Pt: What a dump! You always have to wait here. Why couldn't you get to me sooner?

Dr: All right, Mr. V, calm down. We have a lot of people waiting tonight.

Pt: Calm down? Who do you think you're talking to?

Dr: Listen, Mr. V, I'm the doctor here and I'm telling you to slow down!

Pt: Don't talk to me like that, punk. I'll fix you like I fixed the guys who jumped me.

THE PHYSICIAN'S REACTION TO HIS PATIENT

Reactions to potentially violent patients may result in actions that are dangerous to both patient and physician. Common reactions are listed below, and are further elucidated by the comments in the right-hand column.

Physician's Reaction	*Comment*
Absence of concern about the patient's behavior	Failure to be worried by a patient who threatens him usually indicates that the physician is ignoring his emotions. This may result from the doctor's feeling that it is cowardly or unprofessional to be frightened by one's patients or that patients never hurt their physicians. It is a way of minimizing the patient's dangerousness in the doctor's mind
Anger and a wish to argue with the patient	It is natural to wish to protect oneself from threats with threatening behavior of one's own. However, counter-aggression is likely to threaten the neutrality of the doctor-patient relationship and to provoke the patient to further aggression
Certainty that the physician is in complete control of the situation	If the doctor is unsure about how to proceed with a patient he may attempt to reassure himself by denying the potential seriousness of the situation. This attitude may prevent the physician from protecting himself from the patient
Fear of the patient	It is natural to be frightened of a threatening patient. Attending to this fear will result in the physician's proceeding cautiously and asking for appropriate assistance

COMMON UNSUCCESSFUL APPROACHES

Potentially violent patients can be very difficult to manage, especially if the physician is not accustomed to working with them. Following are some unsuccessful approaches, with the patient's response and an explanation of the patient's behavior.

Physician's Approach	*Patient's Response*	*Explanation*
Tell the patient to stop acting inappropriately	The patient becomes increasingly belligerent	The patient protects himself from feeling powerless, foolish, and frightened by attempting to demonstrate how powerful and frightening he can be. His threatening behavior increases if he feels he is being ridiculed or treated as though he is not frightening
Threaten to call the security guards if the patient does not calm down	The patient threatens to beat up the security guards, too	Since acting belligerent is a way of proving his importance and power, the patient responds to this challenge with increased proof of his manhood
Ignore the patient and continue suturing	The patient's threats become louder and more provocative	The patient's feeling of unimportance increases when he is ignored, and his behavior worsens in an attempt to gain the doctor's attention. He is also frightened by the physician's failure to provide controls and he escalates his behavior to see if the doctor will control it
The physician and one orderly attempt to restrain the patient	The patient attacks them both	The patient feels threatened by the physician's assault and defends himself. He is insulted by the implication that it would only take two people to restrain him, and demonstrates his prowess to them

A SUCCESSFUL APPROACH

If the physician pays attention to his reaction to the patient, he will feel appropriately cautious and take steps to protect himself. This requires that a sufficient number of security guards or orderlies be present to restrain the patient if necessary without injury to anyone and to reassure the patient that he is being taken seriously. With the security force outside the room, the physician is ready to approach the patient safely:

Dr: You seem upset.

Pt: I'm not upset! Why should I be upset?

Dr: Well, for one thing, you've got quite a cut there.

Pt: Damn right...but you should see the other guys.

Dr: What happened?

Pt: I was having a drink and a couple of guys started an argument. Next thing I knew I had to defend myself. But I really put up a good fight.

Dr: You must be very tough, especially since you can talk to me so calmly about your injury.

Pt: It takes a lot of strength to control yourself.

Once the physician feels safe, there is no need to reassure himself by ignoring or arguing with the patient. He can then bolster the patient's self-esteem by acknowledging his power and praising him for controlling himself. When the patient feels that he has gained the doctor's respect, his need to prove himself by frightening the doctor decreases. The physician should then follow these general guidelines:

1. Do not see the patient alone. The physician should always feel completely safe when talking to a patient. Health care professionals should never place themselves in danger.

2. Avoid standing too close to the patient. Belligerent people need increased "body space", the violation of which feels like an attack.

3. Keep the door open.

4. Allow unobstructed access to the door for both physician
    and patient. Both parties should be able to feel that
    they can leave the room immediately if the situation
    becomes dangerous.

5. Do not sit behind a desk or otherwise compromise the
    ability to get away from the patient.

6. Do not see the patient if he has a weapon. A surprisingly
    large number of patients walk into emergency rooms carrying
    concealed weapons. Ask about these and have security guards
    confiscate any weapons immediately.

7. Do not hesitate to call the police if the patient becomes
    too threatening. No physician should be expected to
    manage acutely dangerous patients.

8. Do not argue, fight with, or otherwise challenge the
    patient's self-esteem. Instead, attempt to emphasize
    how much strength and will-power it takes for the patient
    to remain calm and cooperative.

9. Do not threaten force unless the odds are overwhelmingly
    in the doctor's favor. Then, provide a sufficient number
    of burly attendants to subdue the patient safely.

10. Never attempt to subdue the patient alone or otherwise
    be a hero.

11. Discontinue the interview immediately if the patient becomes
    more threatening or the physician's feeling of discomfort
    increases.

12. If a hospitalized patient suddenly becomes threatening or
    belligerent, consider the possibility of an acute organic
    brain syndrome and treat accordingly (see pp. 80-114).

13. If a hospitalized patient without an OBS continues to act
    in a belligerent manner after the guidelines outlined above
    have been followed, inform him that such behavior cannot be
    tolerated in a hospital. If he continues to threaten ward
    staff, obtain a psychiatric consultation. If he needs
    continued inpatient care, arrange for round-the-clock
    attendants or guards or transfer him to a closed facility
    (e.g., psychiatric or prison ward).

EVALUATION OF THE RISK OF VIOLENCE

Whether or not dangerous behavior is the presenting complaint, patients may be encountered whose dangerousness must be evaluated before they can be permitted to leave the emergency room or office. The following factors increase a patient's potential for violence and should be inquired about when dangerousness is a possibility:

1. Past history of violence, including fighting, violent crimes or murder, including killing a soldier of the same or opposite side while in the military

2. Past history of any impulsive behavior

3. Childhood history of cruelty to animals

4. Childhood history of witnessing or experiencing violence or neglect

5. Past history of self-mutilation or self-destructive behavior (which often coexist with homicidal thoughts and acts)

6. Poor job or school record, or other signs of leading a disorganized life

7. History of drug or alcohol abuse

8. Thoughts of injuring or killing someone especially with a specific plan to kill a particular victim that can be carried out

9. Presence of psychosis, especially if voices tell the patient to hurt someone else (command hallucinations)

10. A potential victim (usually a relative or friend) who provokes the patient to violence, e.g., a wife who responds to her husband's threat to kill her with, "you haven't got the nerve"

11. The patient makes the doctor feel frightened or uneasy, and this feeling persists during their interaction

EMERGENCY TREATMENT

If violence is even a remote possibility, the following procedures should be observed:

1. Obtain immediate psychiatric consultation

2. Obtain a thorough history from family and friends

3. Involve family members and other significant people in the treatment from the beginning. Look for covert family provocation or collusion

4. Protect patient and victim by separating them

5. If weapons are an issue, have the patient surrender them immediately

6. Delineate the current crisis and explore non-violent solutions with the patient and his family

7. If the patient remains belligerent, consider the use of medications and/or restraints

8. If the danger of violence remains high, hospitalize the patient either voluntarily or against his will

9. Rule out organic brain syndrome

10. If the patient is allowed to leave, ensure that the patient and his family fully understand and agree with the treatment plan (e.g., a mental health referral), and that the doctor has a way of ascertaining that the patient has followed through

11. Always follow-up on any dangerous patient

APPROACH TO MEDICATIONS

Tranquilizers can be useful adjuncts for calming agitated patients. They are utilized when psychological approaches are unsuccessful, or when there is no time to institute them. Except in abstinence syndromes, medications should be withheld for as long as possible if the patient is suffering from an organic brain syndrome of unknown etiology.

Guidelines for the emergency administration of medications for agitation include:

1. If possible, administer a test dose of a small amount of medication (e.g., 25 mg of chlorpromazine) before administering a therapeutic dose, and observe for adverse effects (e.g., postural hypotension)

2. Offer the patient an oral medication, and allow him a few minutes to decide to take the drug if he does not wish to take it immediately

3. If the patient refuses medication orally, offer it in injectable form. If the patient refuses an injection, let him know that he will be restrained and given the medication if necessary. If he still refuses, restrain him and give the medication by injection

4. Monitor closely patients who receive large doses of medication

5. Use lower doses in older patients or patients with decreased brain function

SELECTION OF A TRANQUILIZING MEDICATION

Five conditions requiring emergency tranquilization are commonly encountered:

1. Acute agitation in which it is not clear whether organic brain disease or a functional disorder is present. Most tranquilizing medications can cause confusion and excitement

in patients with OBS, making diagnosis more difficult. They should therefore be avoided if possible when the diagnosis is not clear. If a medication is necessary, one of the following may be used:

- Paraldehyde 10 cc p.o. or i.m. q 3-4 hrs. until the patient is calm

- Diazepam 5-10 mg p.o. or i.v. q 1 hr. until the patient is sedated. When administered intravenously this drug must be given very slowly or it may cause respiratory arrest. If confusion or agitation worsen, discontinue immediately

- Haloperidol 0.5-3 mg p.o. or i.m. q 1-3 hrs. until the patient is calm

2. Anticholinergic delirium (atropine psychosis). This acute organic brain syndrome is usually caused by scopolamine - containing over-the-counter drugs such as sleeping medications and cold preparations. It is accompanied by dry, flushed skin, dilated pupils, tachycardia, decreased bowel sounds, and fever. Atropine psychosis usually resolves quickly with supportive measures. Extreme agitation or hyperpyrexia are treated with 1-3 mg of physostymine i.v. every 30-60 minutes.

3. Acute agitation definitely not due to organic brain disease. One of the following drugs may be useful:

- Haloperidol 3-5 mg i.m. q 1 hr. until the patient is calm. Acute dystonic reactions may occur

- Chlorpromazine 50-100 mg p.o. or 25-50 mg i.m. every hour until the patient is sedated. The patient should be observed closely for postural hypotension

- Sodium pentothal or amobarbital 100-500 mg i.m. or i.v. until the patient is sedated. These drugs may cause severe respiratory depression and hypotension, and should be administered slowly. They are contra-indicated for patients who may have intracranial disease, hypersensitivity to the drug or porphyria

4. Acute anxiety not accompanied by severe agitation. This may be treated with the following drugs, with follow-up appointments to determine the source of the anxiety:

- Diazepam 5-10 mg p.o. followed by 5-15 mg per day given in divided dose or as an h.s. dose for a few days

- Chlordiazepoxide 10-25 mg p.o. followed by 30-75 mg per day, in divided dose or as an h.s. dose for a few days

- Other benzodiazepines also may be administered short-term

5. Chronic organic brain syndrome (dementia) with episodic agitation. This condition often is encountered in older patients in or outside of institutions. Any nonsedating antipsychotic drug (see p. 250) in low dose may be used, for example:

- Haloperidol 0.5-1 mg p.o. or i.m. immediately and one to three times per day, preferably coinciding with periods of agitation. Extrapyramidal reactions are especially likely to occur in older patients

USE OF PHYSICAL RESTRAINTS

Occasionally, attempts by the physician and his family to calm an agitated patient are unsuccessful, as are the medications described in the previous section. At these times, a sufficient number of orderlies or security guards should be called to demonstrate to the patient that he can be restrained if necessary. This demonstration of superior numbers may allow the patient to calm down without losing face. If the patient's agitation or belligerence continues, physical restraints may be needed. The following steps should then be taken:

1. Do not attempt to restrain a patient without adequate assistance: the physician should never place his own life or safety in danger to subdue a patient

2. Tell the patient that he is being restrained because he is unable to control himself and might injure himself or someone else

3. Explain the procedure to the patient in advance

4. Assign at least one person to each limb. A fifth person can coordinate the procedure. Place one limb at a time into restraints

5. Avoid being kicked or bitten

6. Use leather arm and leg restraints. Body restraints may
    result in strangulation

7. Once the patient is in restraints, place him near the
    nurses' station and <u>check him frequently</u>

8. If there is any danger that the patient may vomit
    (e.g. intoxications, withdrawal states) the patient
    must not be restrained on his back since the danger
    of aspiration is high

9. If the patient continues to struggle once he is restrained,
    sedate him. Continued intense muscular exertion may cause
    myoglobinuria and renal damage

APPROACH TO INVOLUNTARY HOSPITALIZATION

Treatment for patients who are in imminent danger of hurting themselves or someone else or who are severely disabled by a psychiatric
illness can only be provided in a hospital. However, if the patient's
judgment is impaired by his illness or if he cannot bring himself to
admit to the need for hospitalization, he may refuse the care that he
obviously needs. Such patients may need to be hospitalized against
their wills. The following guidelines are helpful:

1. Firmly tell the patient that his condition is serious
    and that it is imperative that he stay in the hospital
    for further treatment

2. If the patient refuses, a temporary mental health hold
    (usually 72 hours) can be obtained

3. Do not attempt to coerce the patient by telling him that
    a hold will be obtained if he refuses to be admitted
    voluntarily. Simply obtaining a hold puts the physician
    on safer ground legally

4. Follow guidelines for restraining the patient if he
    attempts to leave

5. Be familiar with state laws governing involuntary
    hospitalization. Usually, any physician, not just a
    psychiatrist, may obtain a short-term mental health hold

6. Generally, to obtain a hold, the physician should be able to state that, in his opinion, the patient has a mental illness that causes a potential danger to himself or others, or results in grave disability

7. Explain to the patient's family the need for the hold and attempt to enlist their assistance in the procedure

8. Document in writing all behaviors and statements by the patient which indicate the need for a mental health hold. Pay particular attention to suicidal or homicidal threats and behavior that indicates that a mental illness may be present

9. Obtain immediate psychiatric and legal consultation

10. Ensure that the patient has an opportunity to speak with an attorney after he is admitted

11. The chance of a successful lawsuit is slight if, in the physician's best judgment, the patient needs involuntary hospitalization, even if this opinion is not subsequently upheld. On the other hand the doctor may be liable if he does not protect a mentally ill patient who later kills himself or someone else

SUICIDE

Suicide potential should be evaluated in all patients who are upset or who seem depressed. Five to 15% of depressed patients kill themselves, and the suicide rate is high among schizophrenics and substance abusers, too. Although the risk factors listed on pp are useful, even young children have been known to kill themselves and each patient must be evaluated individually. The majority of successful suicides see their physicians shortly before their deaths, at which time they give some subtle clue to their intentions. Physicians (especially house officers) often encounter suicidal patients in the emergency room after they have made a suicide attempt or before an attempt when patients present with vague somatic complaints or other signs of distress.

A TYPICAL PATIENT

A 45-year-old widowed woman complained to her physician of depression and insomnia. She was given a two-week supply of a sleeping medication and a follow-up appointment was made. The next day she is brought to the emergency room comatose after an overdose of the medications.

THE PHYSICIAN'S REACTION TO HIS PATIENT

Patients who have made a suicide attempt often arrive in the emergency room in the middle of the night while the doctor is occupied with other critically ill patients who have not contributed actively to their illnesses. This results in a number of strong reactions, upon which the doctor is especially likely to act if he is rushed. Some common reactions to patients who have just made a suicide attempt are listed below, opposite comments on the doctor's reaction.

Physician's Reaction	*Comment*
Feeling that the patient is wasting the doctor's time when people who are "really" sick need him	Because the suicidal patient often feels angry and helpless, he is likely to evoke similar feelings in the physician. The doctor avoids feeling helpless by dismissing the patient's condition as one with which he should not be concerned. His anger at the patient's behavior then seems justifiable
Conclusion that, since the patient did not kill herself or only made a mild attempt she was not serious about wanting to die	If the physician does not know how to treat the patient or does not like her, he may attempt to avoid her by insisting that she is not seriously suicidal and therefore not appropriate for treatment in the Emergency Room. The patient may then be discharged after a cursory examination, only to be re-admitted later after a much more serious attempt

Physician's Reaction	*Comment*
Wondering why the patient did not do the job right in the first place	Such thinly veiled hostility toward the patient may occur if the physician feels helpless and frustrated, or is responding to the patient's anger (which often is covert). It may result in the physician's encouraging the patient to "do a better job next time"

COMMON UNSUCCESSFUL APPROACHES

Suicidal patients usually feel isolated, misunderstood, hopeless and unable to ask for help. Interventions resulting from a rushed attempt to get them out of the emergency room often increase these feelings, resulting in a subsequent successful suicide. Most attempts to treat medical complications and discharge the patient before evaluating suicide potential thoroughly result from anger at the patient or uncertainty about how to help him.

A SUCCESSFUL APPROACH

Suicidal patients' complaining, demanding attitude and their rejection of offers of help can be extremely frustrating. If the physician remains calm and professional, the following steps can be taken to control the immediate situation and begin thorough suicide evaluation:

1. Place the patient under <u>constant surveillance</u> if any danger exists of his leaving the emergency room before the evaluation can be completed

2. Tell the patient that even though he may be feeling hopeless, his <u>problem can be understood and a better solution found</u>

3. If the patient's <u>family</u> is not present, have them come to the emergency room immediately

4. Obtain a history of the <u>events leading up to the suicide attempt</u>

The physician must then evaluate the continuing immediate danger to the patient's life. The following guidelines will aid in this evaluation:

1. Is the patient glad to be alive? Does he have hope for the future? If not, the risk of another suicide attempt is great

2. Did the patient think that he would be rescued? The patient who did not expect to be saved and did not take steps to ensure rescue is at greater risk

3. Did the patient believe that his method was lethal? The patient who thought that he would die, regardless of the actual danger of his attempt, presents a higher suicide risk

4. Is the precipitating crisis resolved, e.g., did the boyfriend or girlfriend come back, or are conditions the same as before? The patient who returns to the situation that precipitated the attempt may try to kill himself again

5. Does the patient say that he will attempt suicide again? If so, he is likely to do so, especially if he has a plan in mind

6. Do family members indicate a covert wish that the patient die? Comments such as "Why doesn't he get it over with?" indicate such wishes, which may result in the patient's being provoked to make another attempt

7. Does the patient fall into a high risk group? Risk factors as outlined on p. 37

8. Does the doctor feel that the patient might make another attempt regardless of what he says? The physician's intuition should be attended to carefully

EMERGENCY TREATMENT

Most patients entertain some wish not to die even if they make an extremely serious attempt. In addition, even when suicide has been planned for months, the actual impulse to act on the plan usually lasts for minutes to hours, or at most a few days. If the patient can be prevented from killing himself, the immediate danger of suicide is likely to pass. Emergency treatment therefore depends on protecting the patient until he can find other, less lethal, solutions to his difficulties. Ongoing treatment of the suicidal patient should be performed by the psychiatrist. Until a disposition is arranged, the following guidelines should be followed

1. Protect the patient. This may require consistent surveillance or even restraint if the risk of suicide is still high

2. Obtain psychiatric consultation as quickly as possible

3. If the physician decides, after consultation with a psychiatrist, to send the patient home from the emergency room, he should evaluate how reliable the family will be in looking after the patient. This evaluation requires that the family be seen along with the patient

4. If there is any question about the ability of the patient and his family to prevent another suicide attempt, the patient should be hospitalized under 24-hour surveillance. If psychiatric hospitalization is unavailable, hospitalization on a medical floor with a round-the-clock private duty nurse is indicated until transfer to a psychiatric ward can be arranged. Patients have been known to kill themselves even while on psychiatric wards

CHILD ABUSE

Child abuse occurs in all strata of society in patients with all psychiatric diagnoses. At least half a million children are significantly injured each year. Many more are seriously emotionally abused or neglected. Abuse should be suspected when a child is brought to a physician because of repeated trauma, trauma in various stages of

healing, failure to thrive, or unexplained bruising, or when any
suspicious or changeable history of a child's illness is obtained.
Some abusive parents may come to their physicians with vague somatic
complaints, and only reveal the problem when the physician asks about it.

Parents who abuse their children usually have been abused themselves as children. They are frequently distrustful, isolated people
who do not share their feelings easily with others. They have the
unrealistic expectation that the child will meet their needs for love
and appreciation, and become enraged when the child does not meet this
expectation. They usually feel extremely guilty about their behavior
and are therefore very sensitive to criticism.

One child is sometimes singled out as the one who is abused, often
because the parents think of him as different or bad. The child may
have been unwanted, have a congenital anomaly, or remind the parents of
one of their siblings or of themselves. Sometimes, abused children
learn to provoke their parents to anger in overt or covert ways.

The major impediment in identifying child abuse is the unwillingness
of health care professionals to identify the problem in their parents.
Frequently "same-class" bias interferes with this recognition since
physicians are unlikely to look for abuse and neglect in people who
are like themselves. Other physicians do not ask about child abuse
because of overpowering feelings about this problem or because they do
not believe it is treatable.

ENCOUNTER WITH A TYPICAL PATIENT

A mother of two young children complains of back pain, anxiety and
depression. As part of the routine workup, the doctor asks the
patient about her home life. When she seems to dwell on how upset she
is with her children, he questions her more closely about her relationship with them. She reveals that she has been sedating them regularly
with phenobarbital to keep them from making trouble, and is experiencing
frequent thoughts of wanting to beat them.

THE PHYSICIAN'S REACTION TO HIS PATIENT

Child abuse arouses extremely strong negative feelings which often affect the doctor's ability to relate comfortably to the patient. Some of these reactions are listed in the left-hand column below. The right-hand column comments on the reaction.

Physician's Reaction	*Comment*
Inability to believe that a parent would hurt his children	The thought of a child being beaten is upsetting and frightening to most people. To avoid these feelings the physician may conclude that abuse is not a possibility so that he does not need to find out about it
Disgust with a grown person who would hurt a little child	It is understandable that a compassionate adult would object to a child being injured by his parents. This often results in great emotional distance between doctor and patient which the patient, who already is disgusted with himself, senses and responds to by failing to disclose any more information
Conviction that the child must be doing something that warrants punishment	An attempt to excuse the parents' behavior and therefore avoid dealing with it may lead the physician to attempt to see it as acceptable or justified
Temptation to invite the parents to pick on someone their own size	Anger at an abusing parent is especially likely if the doctor identifies with, and wishes to protect, the helpless child

COMMON UNSUCCESSFUL APPROACHES

Many physicians find it difficult to avoid criticizing abusing parents and insisting that if they cared about their children they would stop abusing them immediately. Since the parents already feel guilty and inadequate as parents, and have great difficulty controlling their impulses, these suggestions are likely only to increase their anxiety and guilt and with it, their battering. Other physicians do their best to ignore the problem. The abusive parent's reluctance to confront his problems and his difficulty controlling his impulses make his behavior likely to continue if the physician does not investigate the possibility of abuse and institute appropriate measures to help abusive parents to deal more constructively with their children.

A SUCCESSFUL APPROACH

The definitive treatment of child abuse is carried out by a team of specialists that includes psychiatrists, psychologists, social workers, and paramedical personnel (child protection teams). However, it is often the parents' or the child's physician who first diagnoses the condition. When child abuse is a possibility, the physician should attempt to:

1. Maintain an understanding, non-judgmental attitude

2. Evaluate the entire family

The following questions are useful in investigating the possibility that a patient is an abusing parent. These questions explore bonding and attachment behavior, which is usually warped in abuse and neglect. They may be introduced by asking the patient a general question, such as, "How are things going with the children?"

1. <u>Was the child the result of a planned pregnancy?</u>
    Did the parents make adequate preparations for the
    child? What did they expect the child to be like?

2. <u>What are parental expectations of the child?</u> Is the
    child supposed to be perfect or take care of the parent?

3. <u>Do the children get on the parent's nerves?</u> Few
    parents are never irritated by their children, and the
    parent who denies this completely may be attempting to
    minimize the degree to which his children upset him.

4. <u>What do the parents do if the child is naughty or cries?</u>
    Inquire specifically about the ways in which the parent
    punishes the child, paying particular attention to
    harsh or unusual punishments.

5. <u>Has the parent ever had thoughts of hurting the child?</u>
    Ask him to describe his thoughts in detail.

6. <u>Has the parent ever hurt the child?</u> If so, how badly
    and how often? Have injuries severe enough to require
    hospitalization or broken bones occurred?

7. <u>Can a current crisis in the family be delineated?</u> Even
    an apparently inconsequential problem, such as the
    break-down of a television for a mother who uses it as
    a babysitter, may exceed the capacity of the parents
    to cope with it and result in abusive behavior.

8. <u>Does the parent have a history of being abused as a
    child?</u> Abusing parents are likely to have been abused
    when they were children. Frequently they do not call
    it "abuse" since they feel that they deserved all the
    punishment they got.

EMERGENCY TREATMENT

If abuse is suspected or proved, parent and child must be
protected immediately. The following steps should be considered:

1. Call the child protection team or psychiatric consultant immediately

2. Have the children evaluated by a pediatrician for signs of abuse and neglect. A trauma x-ray screen may be necessary to look for fractures in various stages of healing

3. If abuse is thought to be imminent, hospitalize the abused child voluntarily or against the parent's will

4. Consider hospitalizing the parent(s) since suicide or other violence is a strong possibility

5. If the parent refuses to wait in the office or emergency room until consultation is obtained, follow guidelines for restraining patients (pp. 266-267). If the parent leaves, call the police and child protection team

6. Report all cases of suspected abuse and neglect to the appropriate authorities, usually the local child welfare agencies (this is required by law in most states)

7. Follow-up the case to see what action, if any, has been taken

INCEST

At least 200,000 cases of incest occur each year. Father-daughter incest is the most commonly reported type of sexual abuse. Up to 90% of instances are not reported, however, especially in the middle and upper classes. Incest is found not only in chaotic, disorganized families, but also among those who, on the surface, appear normal. Father-daughter incest, about which the most is known, may occur when the mother abrogates her position and the daughter takes her place. This distortion in family roles, and the incest itself, usually are not apparent to the physician.

Although most family members know that incest is occurring, few say or do anything about it, preferring to keep "peace at any price." The parent who is not directly involved in the incest invariably condones the behavior, at least covertly. The physician, therefore,

must inquire directly about the possibility of incest when the
following clues are present:

1. A young daughter has assumed a central female role in
    the family

2. Perineal or vaginal trauma have occurred at any age

3. Adolescent turmoil and antisocial behavior occur. Fifty
    percent of female runaways give sexual molestation as a
    reason for leaving home. Adolescent suicide also may be
    associated with incest

4. Vague somatic complaints and frequent visits to doctors
    or school nurses in children and adolescents

5. Teenage pregnancy or venereal disease

ENCOUNTER WITH A TYPICAL PATIENT

A respected banker and community leader brings his 13 year-old
daughter to their family physician because she has a vaginal infection.
The father tells the doctor that he cannot understand why his daughter
developed an infection since she is not sexually active. The daughter
says nothing. Two years later, following an abortion and suicide
attempt, the daughter confesses to her physician that her father has
been having intercourse with her and her younger sister for years.

THE PHYSICIAN'S REACTION TO HIS PATIENT

The existence of incest usually is minimized or denied by everyone,
including physicians. Even when the patient confesses, the doctor may
wonder whether to believe her. Other common reactions are described
below, along with comments that elucidate them.

Physician's Reaction	*Comment*
Disbelief that incest could occur in a middle or upper-class family	A wish to deny the problem may lead the physician to believe that it could not occur. However, incest is not confined to lower-class families
Outrage and disgust	Although it is understandable that the physician would be shocked to learn that incest has occurred, he should avoid a punitive attitude that might interfere with history taking or treatment
Conviction that the child is imagining the problem	Contrary to the popular psychological wisdom of a few years ago, it is now known that children tend to under- and not over-estimate sexual abuse. Their reports therefore should be taken seriously

COMMON UNSUCCESSFUL APPROACHES

Because the thought of incest is so upsetting, some physicians may ignore the problem, hoping that the problem will resolve itself. Other doctors openly express criticism of one or both parents' behavior. Both of these approaches lead to a therapeutic stalemate in which the problem is not uncovered or not treated.

A SUCCESSFUL APPROACH

EVALUATION

The physician plays a critical role in the early identification and emergency treatment of incest. Once the problem has been clarified, definitive treatment is carried out by mental health professionals. In addition, since 30% of incestuous fathers turn to the next youngest daughter when the daughter with whom they are involved sexually is no longer available, suspected cases of incest must be reported to child welfare agencies even if the daughter is out of the home.

If incest is suspected, the following questions should be addressed. The subject may be introduced by asking "is anything going on in the home which you are ashamed or worried about?" Since incest usually is not life-threatening, the necessary information may be obtained over a few closely spaced interviews. Parents and children should be interviewed separately.

1. Has the mother been ill, left the home or in other ways abrogated her maternal position?

2. What is the quality of the parental relationship? Are they getting along well? Were they physically or sexually abused as children (a common experience of incestuous parents)?

3. What are the sleeping arrangements? Is privacy respected in the home? What are the bathing arrangements? How is nudity handled in the home?

4. Does the daughter suffer from any of the clues of incest, e.g., early pregnancy, behavioral disorders, perfectionism, etc.?

5. Has any sexual activity occurred between parent or other adult and a child or between children?

EMERGENCY TREATMENT

When incest is disclosed, family members, especially the parent, may become suicidal. The following guidelines apply when incest has been discovered:

1. Evaluate all family members. Pay attention particularly to the possibility that other family members may be involved in incest with the same or different children.

2. Consider a placement for the child away from the family.

3. Refer the child for psychotherapy separately from the parents. Some of the issues with which she must come to terms are anxiety, fear of punishment, conflicts about disrupting the family and guilt.

4. Evaluate all the children in the family for concurrent sexual or physical abuse.

5. Report all cases of suspected or actual incest to the appropriate child welfare agency. Social agencies often are more successful than individual physicians in obtaining treatment for both parents because they are able to offer individual support for each parent and obtain court ordered treatment.

SPOUSE ABUSE

Spousal violence involves a wide range of behavior including emotional abuse and denegration, physical threats, violence and murder. Even though some sort of violence occurs in about 50% of American families, spousal violence usually is overlooked by physicians, even though they have ample opportunity to intervene.

Spouse abuse is a grown-up version of child abuse and often occurs in adults who were abused as children and who are at risk of injuring their own children. As in child abuse, the abusing spouse often experiences extreme guilt and low self-esteem, while the victim often is heavily dependent on the abuser. Weak, ineffectual depressed men in all social groups may beat their wives, while weak, ineffectual, depressed women are likely to remain with men who beat them. Such women may provoke their husbands and even strike the first blow, although fear of losing the husband's support or love are much more prominent motivations for remaining in an abusive situation than anger or a wish to be hurt. Interestingly, as many wives as husbands kill their spouses, in at least 25% of cases because they fear for their own lives.

Victims of spouse abuse seldom volunteer that they are being abused and may even lie to protect their spouses because they fear either retaliation or being abandoned. The following clues suggest that violence may be occurring in the home:

1.   Trauma of any sort, especially when unlikely explanations are offered for its cause. Trauma of the face, arms, abdomen or repetitive trauma or "accidents" are always suspect

2.   Vague somatic complaints in either perpetrator or victim caused by the anxiety, depression or stress that they are experiencing

3.   Any unusual problems during pregnancy, especially unexplained illnesses or injuries, increased family disputes or turmoil in the children

4.   Threats of violence, which should always be taken seriously (see pp. 257-268)

ENCOUNTER WITH A TYPICAL PATIENT

The 29-year-old pregnant wife of a lawyer comes to her obstetrician because of headaches and insomnia. She explains some facial bruises as being the result of hitting herself "on the refrigerator door." Her doctor asks no further questions. One month later the patient miscarries after "falling down the stairs." Eventually it is learned that her husband had pushed her during one of a particularly violent series of arguments which had been ongoing for years without the knowledge of the physician or any of the couple's friends.

THE PHYSICIAN'S REACTION TO HIS PATIENT

As is true of other disturbing family problems, physicians may wish to ignore spouse abuse rather than attempt to deal with this frightening issue. Reactions that support a wish to avoid recognizing and confronting spouse abuse include feelings that:

1. The physician should not meddle in the patient's home life

2. Abuse is easily explained by masochism, sexism, or other popular conceptualizations (thus freeing the physician from understanding the individual patient)

3. Spouse abuse does not occur in the patient's socioeconomic class

COMMON UNSUCCESSFUL APPROACHES

Ignoring or minimizing violence or failing to take appropriate action in the hope that the problem will resolve itself may result not only in further injury, but in the children's repeating as adults what they saw and experienced as children.

A SUCCESSFUL APPROACH

EVALUATION

The primary physician can play a central role in the early detection and emergency treatment of spousal violence only if he is willing to consider the possibility of its presence. Once this problem is suspected, the following guidelines apply:

1. If violence is suspected, ask directly about it when victim and perpetrator are not together

2. Do not be reassured too readily by initial denials of abuse

3. Evaluate the presence of other factors associated with violence such as weapons, drug and alcohol abuse, suicide, child abuse, and injuries of others (e.g., during barroom brawls)

4. Ask about specifics concerning the violence. For example, were fists or weapons used? Have bones ever been broken?

5. How provocative is the victim? Does she dare the husband to hit her, attack his self-esteem, or otherwise invite an attack

6. Evaluate the victim's social resources. Can she leave the home immediately? Is help available in caring for the children? Parents, friends and "safe houses" may be useful resources

7. Consider the possibility of husband abuse. Although much more rare, physical abuse of husbands by their wives may occur

EMERGENCY TREATMENT

The major goal of emergency treatment is the prevention of further injury or death. This is accomplished using the following guidelines:

1. If the danger of violence is still high after the visit to the doctor (this must be assumed if both partners do not express a strong desire for immediate treatment), separate the couple. Hospitalization may be useful in reducing anger and allowing further evaluation

2. Obtain psychiatric consultation immediately

3. Consider referral of the wife to a woman's shelter, safe-house or other agency specializing in the treatment of spousal violence. Definitive treatment is almost impossible if the wife remains in a home in which she is being beaten

4. Support the wife's decision to leave the home temporarily and find support services to help her financially and with her children

5. Offer psychiatric assistance to the abusing spouse

6. Diagnose underlying psychiatric disorders and current psychosocial stresses. Reducing stress and treating psychiatric illness often lowers the potential for violence

7. Consider a report to the local child welfare agency if there are children in the home who are being exposed to a chaotic or dangerous home environment. This may be necessary even if there is no direct evidence of physical child abuse

8. Since abuse is a chronic, long-standing problem, expect relapses and avoid criticizing either spouse if the problem recurs

RAPE

Physicians encounter victims of rape or attempted rape in the emergency room, where the opportunity exists to modify the emotional sequelae of the attack. About 2/3 of rapes are not reported, and the victim may not reveal the attack until months later, when she consults the primary physician because of vague somatic complaints, anxiety and depression, often with suicidal thoughts.

Rape is a sadistic and brutal event that forces the victim to re-evaluate herself and her place in the world. It is difficult to avoid feeling dishonored, vulnerable, humiliated and disgraced.

The psychological reactions to rape are similar to the phases of adaptation to anxiety. The physician may see the patient during any one of these stages:

1. There is an initial period of <u>denial</u> that may be accompanied by feelings that the patient is not real or that the event did not occur

2. This is followed by a period of <u>emotional disorganization</u> when denial alternates with agitation, fear, insomnia and depression. During this period, the patient struggles to deal with the impact of the attack. She may try many maladaptive (e.g., drug use, suicide) or adaptive solutions to her dilemma

3. As the patient begins to <u>reorganize psychologically</u>, her ability to carry out everyday functions increases. Anxiety, depression, and other symptoms recur periodically when the patient thinks about the attack

THE PHYSICIAN'S REACTION TO THE PATIENT

Physicians are likely to have strong reactions to both the victim and the rapist. Common reactions include feeling that the victim provoked the attack in some way, skepticism that the patient actually was raped, curiosity about the details of the assault, and rage at the rapist. All of these reactions serve to distance the doctor from his patient and to distract him from the fact that the patient has suffered an assault that has evoked terror, rage, shame and helplessness.

APPROACH TO TREATMENT

Once the patient is safe, the doctor can help her to begin to express the intense emotions that were evoked by the assault. The following guidelines are useful in helping the patient to begin to deal with her experience:

1. Place the patient in a <u>quiet room</u>, away from the noise and confusion of the emergency ward

2. Maintain an <u>empathic, non-intrusive attitude</u> that communicates an understanding of the turmoil the patient must be experiencing

3. Where possible, ask the patient if she would prefer a <u>female psychiatrist</u>

4. Gently encourage the patient to <u>ventilate her feelings</u>. Tell her that she will feel more in control of her emotions if she can talk about them

5. If the patient is reluctant to discuss her experience, <u>do not force her to do so</u>. This may feel like another assault on her privacy

6. Avoid <u>off-hand comments</u> that might <u>embarrass</u> the patient

7. The necessary <u>physical examination</u> and laboratory tests represent a further intrusion and should be performed <u>tactfully</u>

8. Have a <u>female</u> in the room when examining the patient

9. Talk with the patient's <u>family and friends</u> about their reaction to the rape, and evaluate their ability to offer support. Explain to them the importance of allowing the patient to talk about her experience

10. Make sure that the patient knows how to obtain <u>legal counsel</u> in addition to police assistance

11. Inform the patient about available <u>community agencies</u> that regularly help rape victims and help her to contact one if she is interested

12. Offer the patient a <u>follow-up appointment</u> at which her adjustment may be monitored. If the patient is so preoccupied that she can barely function, or if she denies any thoughts whatsoever about the assault, difficulty adjusting to the experience should be suspected and psychiatric referral recommended

REFERENCES

Kempe CH: The Battered Child Syndrome. JAMA 1962; 181:105

Litman RG, Faberow NL: Emergency Evaluation of Self-Destructive
   Potentiality. In: Faberow NL, Schneidman ES (ed): The Cry for
   Help. New York, McGraw-Hill, 1961

Shader RI: Manual of Psychiatric Emergencies. Boston, Little Brown,
   1975

Slaby AE, Lieb J, Tancredi LR: Handbook of Psychiatric Emergencies.
   New York, Medical Examination Publishing Co., 1975

Weissberg MP, Dubovsky SL: Assessment of Psychiatric Emergencies
   in Medical Practice. Primary Care 1977; 4:651

INDEX